NHS Dirty Secrets

*Bullying, Cover-ups,
Discrimination, Favouritism,
Whistleblowing*

John England

Contents

ᕲ Preface

S ince its inception, in 1948, millions of peoples' lives have been improved and prolonged by the excellent health treatments offered, free of charge, by Great Britain's National Health Service. The idea that a world class standard of healthcare can be provided to ALL citizens, without the need to pay at the point of service, is a reflection of the British generosity of spirit towards those of all classes and sections of society - in the manner of our national characteristic of fair play and equality - and is a reward to the population for enduring the hardships of two world wars.

The NHS has become such an important feature of the British way of life, that the public will consider a political party's attitude to its preservation as a primary factor in deciding which party to vote for in general elections, thereby making it a key component of political debate. No British political party can win over the electorate, if the NHS is not given priority and protection, second only to national defence. Therein lies the problem.

The importance of our National Health Service, to the public, has made it a political football, such that, when any part of the NHS fails to deliver the service expected, the government of the day will attempt to prevent the news of that failure reaching the public and, when the opposition parties discover the failure, they will draw the attention of the public to it, and will promise, should they subsequently be elected into office, that they will ensure to make the improvements necessary to fix whatever it is that needs fixing.

History has shown that, regardless of which party is in power, the government's default reaction to negative NHS news is to conceal it. The public know this, and the public know that the term to describe such default behaviour is the NHS "cover-up culture". It is this culture that prevents instances of avoidable harm from being properly addressed, and is the key factor in ensuring that patient safety is secondary to political imperatives of the government, and financial gain for NHS officials, such as hospital directors and chief executives, who maintain the cover-up culture, on behalf of the government.

📖   📖   📖   📖   📖

I am an anaesthetic technician, more formally known as an Operating Department Practitioner and, informally, as an "ODP". I prefer to use the term "anaesthetic technician", because that better describes what I do; I make the preparations to ensure the correct breathing and monitoring equipment, gases, drugs, and fluids, necessary for an anaesthetist to induce a surgical patient into the state of anaesthesia (seasoned ODPs will often describe their role as being an anaesthetist's "gofor"). Other anaesthetic technician (ODP) duties include taking part in cardiac arrest events and, in a minor way, assisting anaesthetists in sustaining a patient's normal physiology, during their perioperative experience.

The term "Operating Department Practitioner" was created, in typical government style, to foster the image of a profession where the "practitioner" is an autonomous planner, decision maker, and despatcher of clinical services. By creating such an appealing job title, bureaucrats conjure the image that being an ODP is a significant career choice, and the name, by itself, is enough to draw people to the role – being a "practitioner" certainly sounds good.

In reality, ODPs are at the same professional level as nurses, are similarly bereft of influence and autonomy, suffer the same degree of bullying and abuse, and exist to serve surgeons and anaesthetists. There is nothing "practitionerish" about the job of an ODP.

As a career choice, the ODP's progress, as with nurses, is not based on merit, but is very much determined by who their friends are, and who they socialise with, being sycophants of managers, or having close "personal" relationships with senior doctors. This is unfortunate, because those ODPs with intelligence and ambition rarely get to reach their full potential, and that is a loss to both the NHS, and patients.

📖　📖　📖　📖　📖

The motivation for writing this book stems from my unsuccessful quest to encourage a number of government bodies to respond to my alerts (protected disclosures) concerning various corruption and safety issues, such as fraudulently qualified and drug using operating theatre department staff.

It is because none of those arms of government, including the Office of the Prime Minister, responded to my alerts, other than to redirect me to other government bodies, that I decided to continue my whistleblowing in the only manner left open to me, which was to act counter to the NHS cover-up culture, by exposing the truth about that culture, in the form of a book.

Initially, the main aim of the book was to inform NHS employees, who might be considering taking the whistleblowing route to protecting the public, about what obstacles they are likely to face, and what attacks and threats to their careers they could almost certainly expect, should they proceed with their whistleblowing ventures. Additionally, I expected that information about the whistleblowing experience of an NHS employee would be of interest to those members of the public who might want to better understand the inner workings and machinations of the NHS, and its well established cover-up and bullying culture.

However, as I developed the manuscript, my planned whistleblowing message took a different turn. It was not possible to describe the whistleblowing experience, without also describing the core issues of the NHS cover-up culture - bullying, propaganda, incompetence, and fraud. These core subjects soon subsumed the whistleblowing matter and, although my initial plan was to write about my whistleblowing experience, I recognised that this was something that was mostly of concern to me and fellow whistleblowers and, what were originally peripheral matters, soon became much more interesting and central to the underlying problem of the NHS and its cover-up culture. Consequently, I excised most of my own whistleblowing content, and placed that aside for a future book, leaving behind this work – *NHS Dirty Secrets*.

The purpose of this book is to inform, describe, and illustrate, by example, the true character of the NHS cover-up culture, the effects it has on staff, and its consequences to patient safety. The contents are not completely inclusive of all the types of negative issue which infest the NHS but, instead, focus on the principle factors that determine safety and quality of healthcare service delivery, and the methods that the NHS uses to ensure the cover-up culture is maintained.

For experienced NHS employees, from whatever disciplines, be they clerical, doctors, managers, nurses, pharmacists, porters, or radiographers, there might be little in this book that will be shocking, or difficult to believe - these people will have almost certainly become immune to shocks and surprises about what happens in the NHS. They will, however, learn something about the mechanics of the cover-up culture, particularly with respect to the tactics and tricks used to control and suppress employees, and might benefit even more from gaining an insight into the methods and motivations that managers use in their bullying and favouritism practices.

The reader should note that, although most of this book's subject matter is centred on what happens in NHS hospitals, the content also applies to community settings, such as mental health and care homes - the NHS defensive and cover-up culture is all pervasive.

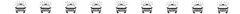

ᕦ Introduction

T he NHS employs thieves, fraudsters, bullies, murderers, incompetents, money launderers, human traffickers, drug addicts, fake doctors and nurses, sexual predators, and other "rogues". Once in a while, information about rogue employees will be uncovered, and evidence will come to light to show that these people have been working against the interests of the public, particularly with respect to patient safety, for a prolonged period. Often, the dangerous or perverse activities of a rogue will have been screened and protected by the NHS cover-up culture, until publicity about their activities forces official action against them. In other words, they have previously been protected by the de-facto "hear no evil, see no evil" policy of the NHS.

Any "rogues", who have not yet been outed, are those who are too discreet to be discovered, or are more deeply protected by the NHS cover-up culture. This cover-up culture, clearly, is in opposition to the intended function of the NHS, which is to improve and preserve the health of patients. The fact that the NHS and its cover-up culture are in opposition is bizarre, but is a reality.

The main aim of *NHS Dirty Secrets* is to describe the NHS cover-up culture, and illustrate how its component parts adversely affect patient safety, the public purse, and employee welfare and numbers.

Emphasis, throughout, is placed on the *Triad of Factors* that constitute the cover-up culture, namely: **propaganda, maskirovka,** and **bullying,** with detailed descriptions of the techniques of propaganda and maskirovka given in appendices 1-3.

The significance of the NHS cover-up culture, to employees, concerns what can happen to them, should they fall victim to bullying, particularly as a management response to them raising issues of patient safety. By appreciating how NHS officials execute the machinations of the cover-up culture, victimised employees might better anticipate, and be less surprised by, the various dirty tricks they can become subject to. This book also helps employees to gain a better understanding of why some people have a "favoured" status, and thrive in the NHS, even though they may not necessarily deserve whatever positive career progress they receive.

For the general public, *NHS Dirty Secrets* can help inform about how and why there are so many well publicised NHS failures and scandals, and explain why their safety, at the hands of NHS professionals, cannot always be assured.

📖 📖 📖 📖 📖

This book has not been written in the style of a single and flowing narrative, instead, it is a combination of narrative, expository, and persuasive styles, where the content is a smorgasbord of issues that are all connected, either directly or indirectly, by the NHS cover-up culture. The reader does not have to progress through the book from start to finish, some people will prefer to go directly to those parts of the book that most interest them, and disregard some of the more dry and technical content. However, for anyone who wants to comprehensively understand the cover-up culture of the NHS, and appreciate the methods that management use to protect that culture, it might be better to read the chapters in sequence, and optionally refer to the Appendices when indicated.

In some parts of the book, readers will notice that sub-sections are quite brief, and text has been replaced with references to websites that provide more detailed information about the relevant subject matter. The reason why these sections are brief is because the original pre-publication manuscript contained nearly one hundred thousand words, which is too much to keep the attention of most people, so, to deliver a book that is a more manageable read, the word count has been reduced to a little more than eighty thousand words.

📖 📖 📖 📖 📖

The first eight chapters describe the NHS cover-up culture, and contain examples of some of the issues that are commonly concealed from the public, and the propaganda and maskirovka (cover-up) methods employed to realise those cover-ups.

Chapter 9 introduces examples of the type of "rogue" people that the NHS employs.

Chapters 10 to 31 are devoted to issues that are mostly concerned with NHS employees, particularly with regard to bullying, cover-ups, discrimination, and favouritism.

The **final two chapters** discuss the subject of whistleblowing, and give examples of how NHS staff have been victimised for raising concerns about patient care.

For readers who might want an in-depth understanding of the

cover-up culture of the NHS, the appendices provide details of the main principles, such as legislation that **should** determine how the NHS functions, plus some of the ways in which it fails to comply with those principles. Also included are explanations of two of the factors that best describe the NHS cover-up culture, specifically, the "rules" of propaganda, and the formal system of concealing truth, known as "maskirovka", which is a topic most familiar to those in political and military circles, but not yet so well known by the general public.

📖　📖　📖　📖　📖

Throughout *NHS Dirty Secrets*, direct mention is made to people, events, and places of work for those issues that are in the public domain, such as the cases that have involved government inquiries. For the less well known matters that I have introduced, hospital names have been aliased with letters of the alphabet to, hopefully, stimulate discussion and exchanges of opinions, amongst NHS employees, about exactly which hospitals I have referred to.

With respect to the names of people whose perverse activities are not yet in the public domain, I have used pseudonyms - for two reasons. Firstly, it would be unfair to directly identify individuals, in a book, where they do not have the opportunity to respond to the accusations made against them.

Secondly, by using pseudonyms, I avoid the possibility of accusations of libel, although it would be unlikely that any of the featured "rogues" would want to draw attention to themselves, in the forum of a civil court, if I did use their real names. Additionally, if any of those "rogues" do want to defend their reputations in court, they would not be able to do so, unless they were prepared to admit that they identified with the particular pseudonym I have assigned to them, and that would be a virtual admission of guilt.

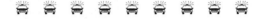

1: NHS COVER-UP CULTURE

"The NHS belongs to the people."

"It is there to improve our health and wellbeing, supporting us to keep mentally and physically well, to get better when we are ill and, when we cannot fully recover, to stay as well as we can, to the end of our lives. It works at the limits of science – bringing the highest levels of human knowledge and skill to save lives and improve health. It touches our lives at times of basic human need, when care and compassion are what matter most."

NHS Constitution - mission statement.

The practice of concealing adverse healthcare issues from the public, particularly avoidable harm, is commonplace in the British NHS, so much so, that the NHS is characterised by its "cover-up culture" - a fact that has been acknowledged by the British Government who, habitually, make exclamations about how they aim to end this culture, because hiding NHS failures is a practice that can deter voters, and losing an NHS related tranche of votes might be enough to lose the government a general election.

The NHS cover-up culture was most publicly highlighted by the Sir Robert Francis "Freedom To Speak Up Review" (2014), which gave recommendations on how to prevent NHS officials from punishing whistleblowers, whose disclosures are meant to serve the public interest, and are a requirement under the *NHS Constitution.*

In reaction to the Francis Report, hospitals produce posters and webpages that encourage staff to raise whatever concerns they have, with the promise that they will not be punished for doing so. Hospitals do this as part of their public relations (propaganda) scheme to deflect from the truth about how whistleblowers are really treated for exposing "cover-ups"; they are punished and bullied and, in some cases, pushed towards suicide.

A useful way to describe the NHS cover-up culture is by considering its purpose and effects. The ultimate **purpose** of the cover-up culture is to protect and promote the image of the government, and its management of the NHS, giving it maximum "votability". The **effects** of the cover-up culture are: low staff morale, high staff turnover, an inexperienced workforce, unsafe staff levels, staff stress, higher levels of sick leave, extra costs of using agency staff, degraded patient safety, and poor public image. It is ironic that the cover-up culture degrades the very public image of the NHS that it is meant to improve - such is the logic of madness.

⚔ Components of a Cover-up

Execution of the NHS cover-up culture is realised by three factors: propaganda, maskirovka, and bullying. The term "**maskirovka**" may be unknown to most readers, because it mostly applies to the advertising, political, and military realms, where concealing information is intrinsic to gaining advantage over an opponent. The NHS cover-up culture cannot function without the application of maskirovka because, otherwise, it would have to rely solely on lies and denial, which are too simplistic and transparent to be very successful. By using maskirovka, the cover-up culture extends to every facet of how the NHS operates, such as employment and promotion of clinical staff who can be relied upon to be loyal to the cover-up culture, because they themselves depend on that same culture, due to them being drug users, fraudulently qualified, or lacking competence for their positions. Perversely, these people who achieve the most job security and career progress. {*Appendix 2 expands on Maskirovka*}.

Propaganda has the purpose of associating positive news with the government, and counter-balances issues that detract from its public image. Law firms, who sell "**Reputation Management**" services to NHS hospital Trusts, protect their clients from scrutiny and sanction, by taking actions that "minimise the negatives, and accentuate the positives", which is propaganda by another name {*Propaganda is covered in Chapter 6 and Appendix 3*}.

Bullying is the process of inflicting psychological damage on the target of a bullying campaign, and is the weapon of choice for attacking anyone who is seen as a threat to the position and status of the bully. Institutional bullying, in the NHS, has the purpose of "removing" threats to the processes of propaganda and maskirovka that enable the NHS cover-up culture to exist, and is the reason why whistleblowers rarely succeed in finding redress to the issues that they raise concerns about – the whole NHS institution is against them, and does whatever it can to suppress and discredit them.

🚑 Cover-up Categories

In the most abstract way, an instance of a "cover-up" can be classed as either "active" or "passive". An **active** cover-up is where effort is made to conceal the absolute truth of a situation, such as using the maskirovka techniques of hiding facts, providing false information (whitewash), diversion, or denial. A **passive** cover-up is the simpler and more effective cover-up category, because it means no news or information is revealed about the matter being concealed – the people concerned just say nothing about the issue.

* * *

To better understand the influence the cover-up culture has on both NHS employees and patients, it is useful to consider what might happen, if the NHS cover-up culture did not exist: efficacy of the patient experience would improve, and there would be fewer instances of avoidable harm to patients, but the increased service transparency would mean that the government would become subject to more public scrutiny, making them less "votable", and that is why the cover-up culture will never be abandoned – the **benefits to the government** outweigh the **costs to patients**.

⛟ 2: MESH IMPLANTS

For readers who do not have direct experience of NHS corrupt practices, it may be difficult to comprehend how the cover-up culture is realised, so, before proceeding further, it might be helpful to set the tone by describing a cover-up model, by using the contemporary example of patients who have suffered harm, due to receiving *mesh implants.*

Surgical mesh is implanted to provide structural support for an organ that has lost some of its integrity, such as when supporting pelvic organs, repaired hernias, reversing prolapse (slippage) of organs as a result of childbirth, and supporting the urethra with Tension-free Vaginal Tape. The idea for mesh implants is not new, it was first postulated in 1890, by a German doctor, Theodor Bilroth, although, at the time, there did not exist suitable methods for implantation, so it was not until 1958 that the first modern implant model was produced, when a mesh made from *polyolefin* was trialled, but proved to be too rigid and heavy to be acceptable by patients. In 1998, a lighter material, mostly polypropylene, was developed, and was quickly adopted world-wide.

Shortly after adoption of this new mesh type, many patients complained that they had started to suffer pain and other problems, such as enteric fistulas (connections between the gastrointestinal tract and other organs), causing pain, nerve damage, incontinence, internal bleeding, and infections. The reason for these problems was found to be the shrinking (1-2%), slippage, and twisting of the mesh, which pressed against, or cut into, surrounding tissues and organs.

The response that affected patients received from doctors and hospitals, about these problems, was denial that the implants were the cause of these new symptoms, and some patients were threatened with legal action, unless they stopped making such vexatious claims. It is worth noting that, although these medical service providers, such as Johnson and Johnson, knew that the implants were causing harm, they refused to halt the practice, because that would have been an indirect admission of the problem and, consequently, that would have opened up the likelihood that mesh sufferers would instigate legal action against them. Given the choice between (1) harming patients and (2) suffering legal action, medical suppliers and providers, invariably, choose to harm patients.

One Canadian sufferer, Chrissy Brajcic, 42, initiated a publicity campaign for victims of mesh implants but, sadly, before she could consolidate her campaign, her implant caused her to develop sepsis, and she died, shortly after.

Subsequent to the publicity of Chrissy's death, the growing number of adverse reports about mesh implants, and the weight of complaints against hospitals, there resulted a general acceptance, in 2018, that mesh implants were the cause of suffering and harm to many patients, and medical institutions, including the NHS, decreed that mesh implantation should only be undertaken as a last resort. In July 2020, incidentally, British Health Secretary, Matt Hancock made a public apology to sufferers of mesh implantation, and promised them recourse of corrective surgery to remove the implants. This acceptance of the mesh problem meant that suffering patients could have their implants removed, and this, indeed, is what has happened.

Unfortunately, the implants have proved to be very difficult to remove and, in many cases, patients have been disingenuously informed, after surgery, that their implants have been completely removed when, in fact, only parts had been removed, with the residual mesh continuing to cause the same debilitating and painful symptoms as were present before "removal".

An illustration of the dishonest and defensive treatment metered out to mesh patients, is that of a London based surgeon, who performs trans-vaginal mesh removal procedures in NHS and private hospitals. This surgeon has a very high success rate with mesh removal, and she has won several awards, and been lauded on television for her successes. However, after claiming successful removal of patients' mesh implants, patients have continued to suffer the same problems they had before the mesh "removal", so some of those sufferers have been forced to seek radiographic evidence of the removal of all mesh, only to be subject to the protective forces of the medical "old boy network", where consultants cover up for each other, and the radiographic proof is falsified, to make it appear that all of the mesh has, indeed, been successfully removed when, in fact, little or none of the mesh has been removed. The evidence for this corruption is in patients consulting diagnostic medical services in other countries, such as the USA, where conclusive evidence for failed removal of mesh implants has been proven. The affected patients were lied to, both by the NHS, and by private hospitals.

Could it be that this (and other) surgeon's success is all a result of self promotion and fraudulent boasting? Indeed it is. Her colleagues know it, and so do the hospitals she works for, but nobody dare speak out, because many would be accused of racism against the surgeon, who is African, and their careers would be destroyed, as a result.

Clearly, promises from the NHS, and government, to address the problems of mesh implants, have been realised with lies, and many patients continue to suffer and face the same, or worse, obstacles that they faced before they underwent mesh removal surgery.

* * *

What this example illustrates is a typical model of a cover-up campaign, that starts with (1) denial of a problem, and which (2) individual sufferers have no power to challenge, because they do not have the financial resources for legal cases to fight their claims. The (3) delay in official acceptance that a problem exists is standard practice, and is part of the process of "passing the buck" that protects officials from involvement in something that might draw negative publicity towards them. It is only when (4) the problem, and its associated adverse publicity, becomes so prolific, that the denials are no longer sustainable, and (5) formal acceptance of the problem is made, (6) an official apology is announced, and (7) the government or NHS promise to make reparations. As is often the case with British governments, their promises to fix a problem, such as this mesh implant issue, are usually platitudes, exemplified by (8) how the NHS has informed patients that their implants have been completely removed when, in reality, they have only experienced partial removals and (9) patients have continued to suffer. In simple terms, the above example of an NHS cover-up campaign for a widespread problem might be condensed into:

Harm - Deny - Delay - Threaten – Evidence overwhelming -

Apology – Promise reparation - Promise not kept

The above simple model of a cover-up campaign is typical for an issue that is experienced by a large group of people, such as mesh victims. However, for an individual patient's issue of avoidable harm, by the NHS, there is no weight of numbers to generate the publicity that might trigger official acceptance that the patient's experience is a real one and, therefore, much less chance that the patient's problem will be addressed, or that they will receive financial compensation for their suffering. Those people suffer alone!

⚑ 3: EXAMPLE COVER-UPS

The following examples give a broad illustration of some of the ways important NHS related issues are concealed from the public. None of the accounts are presented in great detail, because they have only been included to give a flavour of the NHS cover-up culture, rather than being formal reports.

⚑ Ghost Patients

A long established and persistent example of NHS fraud and deception of true facts, is that of "ghost patients", which is the phenomena whereby some General Practitioners have more patients registered with them than the number appearing on the census. According to the *National Institute for Health Research*, "Doctors being paid for 'ghost patients' can be classed as deception and fraud by use of false information". To manage the ghost patient issue, the government relies on the *NHS Counter Fraud Authority* but, because fraud is so widespread, it continues to be a large scale problem, and a significant cost to the taxpayer.

⚑ Unqualified Health Care Practitioners

A growing trend, in the NHS, is to use healthcare assistants to do the work of nurses and allied health professionals (AHPs). These unqualified staff are not subject to national or standardised professional accountability, do not qualify for indemnity insurance, and are burdened with responsibility for patient care beyond their capabilities and training. Patients, of course, are deceived into thinking they are receiving care from qualified staff who are accountable for the care they give.

Hospitals attempt to give the impression that unqualified staff are properly competent, by enrolling them on locally produced training schemes, and sending them on short courses at universities (ex-polytechnics), so that they create the image of professional credibility. These courses are shallow and unsubstantial tick box exercises, which have no academic merit, and do not prove competence or knowledge about the safe delivery of patient care.

After completing these short courses, the unqualified healthcare workers become fraudulently "qualified", with faux qualifications which are meant to deceive, rather than give proof of competency or safety. This scheme is classic behaviour for the NHS, where qualification is not by competence, but by "certificate of competency". Curiously, the public do seem to be convinced by printed "certificates" of qualification, which prove to be very effective at giving credibility to what are commonly referred to as "mickey mouse" qualifications.

Qualified NHS staff, of course, are not convinced by these fake qualifications, and they know the patient safety implications of such practices, but they do not have the freedom to speak out about this or other issues of public concern, because they know they will be bullied and punished for doing so.

♖ Redefining Trolleys as Beds
An infamous NHS example of an ultimately failed deception occurred

in the early 2000s, when there was much publicity about the lack of hospital beds, and the consequent high number of patients being parked on trolleys, in corridors. The NHS responded to this bad publicity by redefining trolleys as beds, if they had their wheels removed. Hospitals then started removing wheels from trolleys, with the result that they were able to report fewer cases of patients on trolleys, and more patients on beds.

This particular issue may be a historical one, but it does accurately exemplify the ongoing attitude that the NHS has regarding bad publicity – the policies and practice of deception and redefining of "facts" are persistent.

⚙ Cancer Patients

A particularly nasty NHS **dirty secret** concerns the manipulation of facts, at hospital T, where patient safety is compromised, in return for the hospital being able to report compliance with a government target which, specifically, concerns cancer screening. At this hospital, patients supply tissue cells that undergo various tests to determine whether or not those cells contain clinical markers, which could indicate early signs of cancer. When those tests prove positive, the hospital is obliged to inform the patient about the test results, and provide them with an appointment for further, more in depth testing. The timing of any ongoing patient communications and testing is determined by government targets, which must be adhered to, otherwise delays in further testing and treatment may result in a worsening of the patient's condition.

In this particular incident, the number of patients requiring follow-up testing exceeded the hospital's capacity to execute those tests within the specified government target dates. To avoid being reprimanded for failing to meet a target, the department manager, David Green (band eight nurse), an enforcer of his department's cover-ups, instructed a clerical worker, who was responsible for composing and posting appointment letters to patients, to delay sending some of the letters until the start of the following month, so that the target for the current month would not be exceeded. The clerical worker was horrified at such a directive from her manager, and refused to comply with his unwritten and unwitnessed instruction, because it had the intention of giving his own status and job security a higher priority than the safety of cancer patients. For her disobedience to the manager, and her disloyalty to the hospital's cover-up policy, the clerical worker was threatened, disciplined (for other reasons), and bullied out of her job – she quit because she was overwhelmed by the bullying campaign inflicted on her.

▣ Hospitals Fail to Investigate Patient Deaths

One Care Quality Commission's (CQC) Chief Inspector of Hospitals, Professor Sir Mike Richards, criticised NHS hospitals for failing to investigate most patient deaths, ignoring relatives of the deceased patients, and excluding them from enquiries into those deaths. According to his 2019 report, the NHS failure to look into the causes of patient deaths is a system-wide problem, which results in the NHS not learning from their mistakes.

Deborah Coles, the director of *Inquest*, an organisation which investigates patient deaths, said the CQC review of how hospitals respond to patient deaths, had exposed "a defensive wall surrounding the NHS, an unwillingness to allow meaningful family involvement in the process, and a refusal to accept accountability for NHS failings in the care of vulnerable patients". (The term "defensive wall" is a synonym for "cover-up culture".)

🕮 Hospitals Fiddling Death Rates

According to a report by healthcare analysts, *Dr Foster Intelligence*, hospitals are "fiddling the figures" on hospital deaths, by increasing the number of deaths recorded as being palliative, which means that the patients were classed as being terminally ill, who were only admitted for pain relief, not for treatment of their conditions. In this way, no investigations into those deaths are deemed necessary, and the relevant hospitals do not attract undue attention for deaths that were avoidable.

One example given, by *Dr Foster Intelligence*, is that of a low risk patient who was admitted for a hip replacement, but unexpectedly died during his admission, so his clinical code was changed to show that he was a palliative patient; by changing his code, the hospital avoided negative publicity which would otherwise accompany any formal Hearing process about the unexpected death.

Clinical coding is not a subject which attracts public attention - it functions below the radar of scrutiny - but, inevitably, it will almost certainly come under forensic analysis, all that is required is a knowledgeable whistleblower to come forward.

🕮 Did Not Attend

The "success" of an NHS hospital is measured by its ability to meet targets, set by government, which uses those targets as propaganda, painted as "proof", that politicians use to convince the public that they are doing a good job of ensuring their optimal medical health, by getting the greatest number of patients through the system. One target, for example, could be the number of a specific type of operation performed in a particular month. If a scheduled patient fails to turn up for that operation, known as a *Did Not Attend* (DNA) event, the "target" count may not be affected, because the hospital was not to blame for the operation failing to be performed. The patient will then be rescheduled, but may be punished for their DNA by being pushed a long way down the waiting list, rather being placed near the top. This means, of course, they will spend more time in pain or discomfort.

To ensure that they meet a target, the hospital can employ a commonly used NHS trick, which is to fraudulently inform the patient, by letter, that they were booked to have their operation but, because they failed to attend (DNA), they will have longer to wait for a new appointment. In this way, the hospital is able to meet the target, and may even exceed it, if that is their aim (bonuses?).

Another version of the fake DNA scam, designed to make it appear the hospital is meeting a target, occurs when a patient turns up for an appointment, but their medical notes record the appointment as being a DNA. This trick seems to be more commonly used with patients who are less likely to recognise what has been written in their notes, either because they have vision problems, do not understand English, or are very elderly.

✍ Pharmacy Screening

An important aspect of patient safety is that which concerns pharmacological screening by the hospital's pharmacists. The purpose of the screening is to determine which drugs are safe for a particular patient, and are appropriate for their ever-changing condition. Such screenings check for allergies, medical history, and effectiveness of medication regimes, so that optimum and safe medical prescribing can be tailored for each patient.

To properly and safely screen a patient, the pharmacist must spend whatever time is necessary to understand an individual patient's condition, including extra time that might be required for foreign language interpretation, or with other communication difficulties. Consequently, it is not possible to allocate an exact period of screening for each patient, so screening time must be allocated according to individual patient needs. The problem is that hospitals will not allow enough time for a pharmacist to properly screen all of the patients who are allocated to them, so they will have to rush the screening process, to meet their specific targets, and that can mean they miss important issues that might degrade patient safety. Predictably, having to meet a target of how many patients are screened, per shift, leads to bullying of pharmacy staff, by management, and compromises the legal duty to reduce risk. If a rushed screening means that safety related patient information is overlooked, and the patient suffers harm as a result, it is the pharmacist who will be held accountable by the NHS blame culture – not the hospital management. By ensuring that the pharmacist is accountable for the patient's drug related safety, managers are able to deflect and cover up their own responsibilities, and the pharmacist has no avenue for resolution of the whole screening regime – either from their registration body, or the NHS.

⏣ Torrington Community Hospital

In the years before announcing their decision to close down Devon Torrington Community Hospital, the regional Clinical Commissioning Group redirected many of the Torrington patients to other hospitals, making it appear that the hospital was not being fully utilised and, therefore, not needed. The regional Clinical Commissioning Group then had justification in closing the hospital, as per its original intention. This is an example of the maskirovka technique of achieving a goal by hiding intentions (to close the hospital) by manufacturing some justification (under utilisation).

⏣ Staff Blunders

In 2015, Jeremy Hunt, Health Secretary, announced that the NHS cover-up culture was concealing at least one thousand unnecessary patient deaths each month, caused by staff mistakes. Mr Hunt's claim that these patient deaths were due to staff mistakes is an easy way to deflect blame from where it belongs which, ultimately, is the Department of Health, onto the obvious scapegoats, who are the frontline NHS staff.

The general public will hear a statement of this sort, that staff are to blame, and take it at face value. Sometimes, staff are to blame, because of incompetence or an uncaring attitude – but staff blunders are not always caused by the staff themselves. Often, when looking a little deeper, it is much more likely that the underlying cause of the problem lies with NHS and Department of Health officialdom, especially in those cases where patient deaths are due to hospitals being understaffed and under resourced, and where staff are persistently bullied into refraining from speaking out about the poor state of patient safety.

The issue of scapegoating frontline staff is not limited to clinical line managers and team leaders, it extends all the way up the chain of command to the government, so it is institutionalised.

♔ Statistical Dirty Tricks

♟ Scheduling Trick

This is when a hospital schedules a patient for a non-emergency operation when being aware that the patient would not be available at that time because, for example, they would be on holiday. This enables the hospital to meet specific targets for patient numbers, and reducing queue figures.

♟ Fake Short Waiting Lists

Hospitals have been found to only add patients to surgical waiting lists during the months they had their operations, so making it appear that waiting lists were very short.

♟ False Reporting

Investigators have also discovered hospitals adjusting clinical treatment details and dates for government reports, so that service delivery figures appeared to be better than they really were.

♟ Golden Goodbyes

Directors and senior managers, who are dismissed for misconduct or incompetence, are given large redundancy payments, then re-hired by the same hospitals, sometimes with six figure "golden hello" payments. This is the NHS "old boy network" in action.

♨ Patient Deaths

♨ Death from Dehydration

In 2009, Kane Gorny (22), a sufferer of *diabetes insipidus*, was admitted to St George's Hospital, Tooting, for a hip replacement operation. During his admission, none of the staff read his medical notes, he was not given fluid balancing medication for his insipidus, and neither his fluid or sodium levels were monitored. As part of his treatment, endocrinology specialists should have been assigned his case, but they were not informed of his admission.

Kane made persistent pleas for a drink of water, but staff ignored his requests so, out of desperation, he called his mother, and the police. When the police arrived, staff sent them away, telling them that there was no need for concern. Kane was not subsequently given water, or fluid balancing medication and, before his mother arrived, he died of cardiac arrest, resulting from dehydration and hypernatraemia (excess sodium).

At his inquest, the Coroner, Dr Radcliffe said: "Kane Gorny died as a result of dehydration, contributed to by neglect. He was undoubtedly let down by the incompetence of staff, poor communication, a lack of leadership, both medical and nursing, and a culture of assumption". After spending some time sitting with his lifeless body, Kane's mother was asked, by a nurse, 'Have you finished? Can I bag him up now?' (the nurse's lack of sensitivity is not uncommon in NHS hospitals).

This case might be considered too old to be relevant today, but Kane's death did not result in improved protocols, staff training or any other mitigating steps designed to prevent recurrences of the mistreatment he suffered. Moreover, St George's still employ staff whose qualifications are not validated, and who are not properly screened and tested for their knowledge, abilities, or attitudes.

♞ Glasgow Child Poisonings

After a child patient died, in 2017, from the contaminated water supply of the *Glasgow Queen Elizabeth University Royal Hospital for Children*, Labour Member of the Scottish Parliament, Anas Sarwar, accused Scottish NHS officials of covering up the death. Earlier investigations discovered that the water supply had caused twenty-six child patients to be infected with the stenotrophomonas bacteria. Mr Sarwar claimed this matter was being hidden from the parents, politicians, and the public.

▰ Patient Advice and Liaison Service

The purpose of a hospital's PALS office is to provide patients with information regarding the services they can expect from the NHS, and confidential advice concerning any complaints they want to make about the service or treatment they have been subjected to. For minor matters, PALS is a very useful resource to use but, for serious matters, such as medical negligence, consulting with PALS is inadvisable. The reason for that is because the underlying function of PALS is not to help patients, but to protect the hospital from any possibility of legal sanction, or any matter that might attract bad publicity for the hospital, Chief Executive, or the NHS in general. Many victims of poor treatment, or avoidable harm, will automatically use the PALS service as the first point of contact for making complaints, thinking that PALS will advise them on how to best proceed with the formal complaint process, but this is not what happens. Instead, PALS will use the techniques of denial, obfuscation, and anything else that will prevent the complaint from being accepted as valid, so that the hospital does not accept liability.

For complaints about clinical care, the best course of action is to seek advice from a solicitor who specialises in medical negligence cases. If the solicitor recommends lodging a formal complaint with the hospital's PALS office, then that advice should be taken. However, when making the complaint, it should be made in writing, and the complaint should only include whatever information is approved by the solicitor. Complaints should not be made in face-to-face meetings with PALS staff, because that opens up the possibility of PALS making false allegations, such as aggression, against you, the complainer (plaintiff), and that could lower the chance of reaching an acceptable resolution to the complaint. Another reason for avoiding spoken dialogue with PALS is due to the strong possibility of your conversation being covertly recorded, and the trickery from experienced PALS officers might well draw you, the complainer, into revealing information that you would be best keeping to yourself, particularly with respect to whatever next steps you plan to take. They might also provoke you into anger, and that would then make you vulnerable to accusations af aggression, with the result that the focus moves from your clinical issue to your character (*tone policing*).

Most significantly, as with anything else concerning the NHS, do not assume that the information you share will be treated as confidential, because it won't be. Remember, regardless of what the hospital literature and posters say, PALS staff are not there to help patients, they are employed, ultimately, to protect the hospital chief executive's position, and the reputation of the hospital, so do not trust them!

♨ Investigation Procedures

♨ Risk Reduction

Members of the public might assume that, when a patient dies, unexpectedly, the NHS would have systems in place to ensure that independent and impartial inspectors are sent to discover the cause of the death. Then, if those investigators discover that the death was preventable, and caused by systemic or individual failures, then they would ensure that mitigating actions are taken to reduce the probability of a repetition of the incident, and the information about the case would be propagated to other parts of the NHS, so that lessons would be learnt throughout the organisation, with the result that preventative measures would stop other patients from dying from similar reasons to the patient being investigated.

By being open about the causes of death, and taking risk reducing measures, the NHS would comply with the *Health and Safety at Work Act*, obligation to reduce risk. Unfortunately, such openness and legal compliance is not part of NHS behaviour, as many family members of patients who have died unexpectedly, whilst in NHS care, will attest to. What many of these people face is the suite of deception techniques designed to conceal NHS culpability, with denial, false information, and the problem of missing patient records being the main defensive weapons used by NHS officials (to protect their positions).

♣ Missing Patient Records

Social media reports of hospitals avoiding culpability for patient deaths, by "losing" or editing patient records, which might otherwise provide proof of neglect and mistakes, are prolific, to the extent that losing patient records appears to be standard NHS practice. Legally, this practice is known as *Spoliation*.

☠ Spoliation

The destruction or alteration of evidence resulting from a party's failure to preserve evidence relevant to a litigation or investigation.

There are three particular aspects of this NHS spoliation that are worthy of note:

1. If a hospital "loses" the care record of a patient who has died, unexpectedly, then that is something that should quite reasonably be reported to, and investigated by, the police. After all, an unexpected death has occurred, and if the cause cannot be discovered, because of missing notes, then there might be no way of learning whether or not the death was due to a Dr Harold Shipman type episode, where the patient is intentionally killed by someone involved in the patient's care pathway. Strangely, the police, in the main, take no interest in deaths of patients in the care of the NHS.

2. Much, if not all, of the information that is contained in patient care records is electronically duplicated on hospital computer systems. These systems, which are formally known as "Management Information Systems" use commercially available software which, typically, are *Oracle* or *Microsft Sql Server* relational database systems. If the paper version of a patient's care record is lost, then that information can be easily reproduced from computer storage, which means that a hospital's excuse that they have lost the patient's records is a deceit. If the hospital were to claim that the computer data has also been lost, then that is another attempt at deception, because all management information systems have automatic duplication and backup systems incorporated into their software "packages", and recovering lost data is not just achievable, it is a standard facility for management information systems.

3. In the early 1990's, the British government incorporated the *Precautionary Principle* into health and safety legislation. The purpose of the Precautionary Principle is to remove any excuses for inaction on the grounds of missing information, or uncertainty. Consequently, when a patient has come to harm, but there is no available evidence, such as might be contained in a patient's notes, to prove that the harm was avoidable, then the Precautionary Principle should be invoked and, by so doing, the assumption should be made that the death was avoidable, and the hospital has failed to prevent the harm.

The spoliation of patient notes, according to the law, should not be used as an excuse to dismiss the plaintiff's patient/family claim that harm to the patient was caused by mistakes or inadequate care, but that is, indeed, what does happen.

♣ Discharging Patients

Every NHS hospital has its own detailed policy for discharging patients, and all have the intention of ensuring their patients have appropriate post-surgery care instructions, drug prescriptions, GP advice details, and can safely travel home. On the whole, discharge nurses ensure these discharge protocols are properly followed. Unfortunately, some hospitals have very sloppy management and control procedures for discharging patients, and safety suffers as a result. One hospital, which has an ongoing reputation for unsafe discharge events, and which features elsewhere in this book, is Pilgrim Hospital in Boston, Linconshire.

At Pilgrim, it is not unusual for elderly or confused patients to be discharged before they have fully recovered from surgery, so that the discharge matron can improve her targets for freeing up beds. Consequently, a patient may be discharged without the nurses arranging for the patient's carers or family members to escort the patient home, so the patient is taken outside, and made to find their way home, on their own. Additionally, the patient may not have been given their "take home" pain control drugs, follow-up treatment instructions, and so on. But, if a patient or carer makes a formal complaint about the discharge process, the patient record will be amended to "prove" that procedures were followed, and that the patient was given their drugs, but must have misplaced them. This is another example of the spoliation process.

♣ Vyaire Enflow Fluid Warmer

When patients undergo surgery for more than thirty minutes, or receive blood administration, their intravenous line will incorporate a fluid warming device, of which the NHS use several types, including the Enflow fluid warming device. The Enflow warmer incorporates a heated aluminium cartridge, over which the administered blood or other fluid flows, to be warmed, before it enters the bloodstream.

In March 2019, the Medicines and Healthcare Regulatory Agency issued a Field Safety Notice (FSCA 19-001), which instructed hospitals to cease using the Enflow system, because they had discovered that it released aluminium, which is toxic, into the bloodstream. The toxic affects of aluminium include: Alzheimer's disease, breast cancer, bone weaknesses, brain diseases, anaemia, seizures, muscle weakness, slurred speech, respiratory problems, nervous system damage, and difficulty in controlling limb movement.

As a consequence of this Safety Notice, hospitals that used the Enflow system should have informed all patients about the alert, and created testing procedures to monitor the ongoing health of those patients. This didn't happen.

Why? Because the NHS does not want to be liable for the extra costs involved in monitoring at risk patients, or to be exposed to the potential for legal sanction for exposing patients to harm. The NHS prioritises protecting itself over protecting patients.

♣ Voluntary Erasure from the General Medical Council

When a patient suffers avoidable harm from a doctor who is near to retirement, that doctor can avoid professional scrutiny and sanction from the General Medical Council, Care Quality Commission, Parliamentary and Health Service Ombudsman, and the NHS, by voluntarily erasing their name from the GMC, and taking early retirement, with full and generous pension entitlement. The patient will then lose all routes to redress, unless they have the finances to take independent legal action, which would involve spending a minimum of one million pounds in solicitor and barrister fees. For most people, that would not be possible, so they would just become casualties of the system, which is a common problem. It is worth noting that the above organisations are all government bodies, whose underlying purpose is to protect the government – not patients.

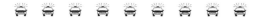

⛟ 4: KILLING OFF OLDER PATIENTS

I n the early 1990's, the British Prime Minister, John Major, was asked why, given the latest evidence proving the dangers of cigarette smoking, was he so disinclined to ban smoking or, at least, to discourage children from taking up the habit. Mr Major's response illustrated his attitude towards the health and quality of life for the populace, by giving two reasons why smoking should not be banned: firstly, he said, smoking results in a lot of valuable tax revenue; secondly, because smoking shortens people's lives, the government saves the money that would otherwise have to be spent on those people living and drawing pensions for longer, and needing more NHS resources, which increase with age. In short, shortening the lives of the elderly helps the government save money so that they are able spend those savings on their pet projects, such as bribing third world despots, under the guise of "aid", in return for political support in international issues.

This penchant for a form of passive and indirect euthanasia was not something that was particularly linked to John Major; far from it, culling the elderly population appears to be a cross party sentiment – MPs, especially Labour, are quick to publically express how important and wonderful are the youth of the country, but positive statements about the elderly are never more than propaganda. Indeed, British politicians seem to take any opportunity to kill off the elderly – disguised by whatever means are convenient for the time.

♣ Motivations and Methods

The philosophy of killing off the elderly is still part of political philosophy, and is another one of the NHS's dirty secrets. Killing off elderly patients helps hospitals to get closer to satisfying government "targets" for patient throughput, and that is of benefit to the job security of hospital Chief Executives, and the general positive image of the NHS and standing government.

♣ Liverpool Care Pathway (LCP)

Worth mentioning is the LCP end of life scheme, which was meant to minimise suffering of terminal patients in their final hours, and realised by denying patients intravenous nutrition and hydration administration (*passive euthanasia*). Predictably, some doctors were over zealous in using the LCP, would not consult with the families of patients, and saw the death of a patient as an easy "care" option. There were also reports, notably by the Daily Telegraph, that hospitals received extra money for each patient who was put on the LCP - stimulated by improving the hospital's targets. The LCP was outlawed in 2014 but, according to many people whose family members have unexpectedly died in hospital, the practice still continues.

♣ Active and passive ways of killing patients

Killing patients can be achieved in both passive and active ways: **Passive** methods refers to denying patients proper care, such as medical treatment, drugs, resuscitation, nutrition, oxygen, hydration, infection control, and pressure sore management. **Active** methods are doing things that directly affect the patient, with the best example being that of administering over-doses of opiate or sedative drugs, whose effects can produce respiratory depression and cardiac arrest. It is worth noting that one of the NHS's most commonly used sedative drugs is a benzodiazepine called *Midazolam,* which is the drug used by some American states when executing prisoners by lethal injection.

The description of this phenomenon can be condensed into the postulation that killing off the elderly helps hospitals meet targets, and helps politicians keep their jobs. Such is the reality of morality in 21st century Great Britain.

♿ Gosport War Memorial Hospital

During the period 1987 – 2001, the lives of more than 600 Gosport War Memorial Hospital patients were shortened by the unnecessary over-dosing with opiate and sedative drugs. It is believed that the number of dead patients to be 200 higher than the 600 reported, but this can't be proved, because their clinical notes have gone "missing".

At the 2018 NHS inquiry into this Gosport hospital found that elderly patients were considered to be nuisances and "bed blockers", and were given continuous drug infusions to "keep them quiet". Many of these patients died within a few days of their admittance to hospital. The inquiry concluded that an intensive care doctor, Dr Barton presided over an "institutionalised regime which had a flagrant disregard for human life".

Between 1990 and 2001, several nurses raised their concerns about the inappropriate drug administration practices, and the disproportionately high number of deaths of elderly patients, due to the habitual over-prescribing by Dr Barton, who staff referred to as "Dr Opiate". Hospital managers ignored the concerns of those nurses which, inevitably, allowed the practice to continue, and facilitated the continued killing of "nuisance" elderly patients. One of the nurses, Sylvia Giffin, who reported her concerns, was bullied out of her job, and suffered depression as a result. She died in 2003.

Prosecutors failed to secure a conviction of murder or manslaughter against Dr Barton. (Cover-up culture?)

⚸ Do Not Attempt Resuscitation (DNAR) Instructions

♣ DNAR defined

A DNAR document, sometimes referred to as DNACPR, or DNR (Do Not Resuscitate), is a signed and witnessed instruction from a Doctor that, should a patient suffer cardiac arrest, no attempt should be made to resuscitate them. In effect, it means that the arresting patient should be allowed to die. The justification for a DNAR instruction is based on the likelihood of success of resuscitation, and whether or not the attempt could cause unreasonable trauma, such as breaking the patient's ribs, during CPR. Attempting resuscitation on a patient who is desperately sick, and is at the end of their natural life, can be a pointless exercise, and will almost certainly extend their suffering, so is not always desirable.

However, a DNAR instruction is not just a Doctor's decision, because the patient may themselves request that they do not receive specific life saving treatments, such as antibiotics, CPR (resuscitation), or ventilation (breathing tube in the windpipe). This is decided by the patient, and witnesses, completing an *Advanced*

Decision to Refuse Treatment document. However, neither the patient, nor their family, can INSIST that resuscitation attempts should be made. The final decision is left with the Doctor, and that decision should be based on the best interests of the patient.

♣ Patient and Family Discussions

When faced with the DNAR problem, patients and their families should be aware of a legal precedent, established in 2014, which states that a Doctor should not make a DNAR decision without involving the patient and their family in the decision process. Unfortunately, a recurring problem, in the NHS, is that of a minority of Doctors signing DNAR forms – without informing the patients or their families of the fact. Doctors should NOT make such arbitrary decisions, but they do. In general, the public do not understand the legal or ethical aspects of DNAR orders, so Doctors get away with it.

♣ Blanket DNAR Addendum

Since first publication of this book (January 2020), another DNAR issue has come to light, during the Covid-19 outbreak, which is that of blanket DNAR instructions being issued to NHS patients and residents of care homes (particularly in North London, South Wales, and Sussex), based on the criteria of mental health, or age which, in some cases, means patients as young as fifty years old.

What issuing blanket DNAR instructions means, in effect, is that the NHS has an unofficial policy of *passive euthanasia* even though, under British law, euthanasia is classed as murder or manslaughter.

Initially, neither the NHS or government made public comment on this issue – it was an "unofficial" practice so, in effect, it was covered up. However, there has been such an avalanche of complaints about blanket DNAR practices, especially on social media (on Twitter, search for "DNAR" or "DNR"), keeping this issue covered up proved to be impossible. Consequently, both the Care Quality Commission and the NHS Medical Director, Professor Stephen Powis, have issued guidance that prohibits the issuance of blanket DNARs. So, it is only because of discovery and complaints from the public, and not action from the community of doctors, that this practice has been officially repudiated – although that does not mean the practice has stopped.

♿ DNAR Analysis

When considering the issue of "allowing" patients to die, through DNAR directives by doctors, the potential user of NHS services might want to ponder the following points and, in particular, recognise that there is no need for evidence to prove that any of the scenarios exist because, following the Precautionary Principle, and the fundamental axiom of Safety and Reliability Engineers that, if an adverse event can happen – it will happen, it has to be presumed that these things do happen. Indeed, if it were to be postulated that, even though doctors can cause or allow patients to die but, because they have strong ethics, they do not do so, that would be both extremely naive, and statistically, virtually impossible. In fact, there is no need to defend the claim that doctors do kill patients, either directly or indirectly, because there is plenty of historical evidence of the fact, both in the UK and elsewhere, such as the case with Jane Barton, Harold Shipman, Josef Mengele, Mohammed Asha, and Muhamed Haneef, to name but a few.

There is also the more contemporaneous issue of racial hatred that has come to the fore of public debate, by the Black Lives Matter organisation, where its members and leaders have expressed their belief that the lives of white, Hispanic, and Asian people do NOT matter. Once again, it would be very, very naive to assume that no BLM supporting doctor, paramedic, nurse, or anaesthetic technician (ODP) would not, by omission or commission, cause the death of a patient whose life they consider to not matter, so, sneaking a DNAR form into a patient's notes is something that should be assumed definitely does happen.

> Of course, this issue of discrimination can apply to people of any race, religion, or belief system. Even as a male English NHS employee, working in England, such discrimination against me, and my fellow English male colleagues, and occasional English female colleague, is all pervading; anti-Englishness is so endemic, it is just taken for granted that every foreigner/immigrant wants to harm your career and social standing. Three foremost examples of racist doctors (anaesthetists) who make no effort to hide their anti-Englishness are Dr Patel (Royal Throat, Nose, and Ear Hospital), Dr Elaine Monahan (St George's Hospital), and a Northwick Park Hospital anaesthetist who is easily identified by his habit wearing "scrub" hats with symbols that include the swastika on them. Each one a highly paid racist yobbo!

As with everything where evidence is systematically hidden from view, it is the Precautionary Principle and rules of probability that dictate whether or not such things happen: if it can happen, it will do!

♣ Motivations for DNAR orders

If a particular ward has 30 beds, all occupied by very sick and/or elderly patients, and there is a growing list of new patients who need some of those beds, the longer the waiting patients spend in the queue for beds, the more likely it is that "targets" for waiting list numbers and times will be breached, and the greater the likelihood that the waiting patients/families will report their concerns to the press. News of the target breach will then make its way to the overseeing Health Authority, and that will impinge on the reputation of the hospital CEO (Chief Executive Officer), and that, itself, might be enough for the CEO to lose their very lucrative and easy (they don't do much) post. CEOs, therefore, ensure that pressure flows down to the front-line doctors to do something to speed up the freeing up of beds, otherwise, quite predictably, the careers of those doctors will be negatively affected by their failures to act in the best interests of their CEOs. There is only one way to free up some of the above beds, and that is to "assist" or "allow" patients to die, and such methods as DNAR, over-sedation, and dehydration (nil by mouth) are the easiest and preferred methods used, particularly when, as a rule, no questions are asked when a patient dies. This is one of the consequences of NHS targets – some patients are a threat to achieving targets and, because those sick patients are a problem that can't be solved, by making them better, the problem itself is removed, by "removing" the patients; all for the benefit of the careers of the doctors concerned, and their CEO.

♣ Laziness

For some doctors, if it might be preferable to issue a patient a DNAR order, rather than actively manage and try to improve the patient's condition, because it is less hassle! Allowing the patient to die is such an easy thing to do, it is low risk, and with rarely any comebacks to the issuing doctor, because they are giving carte blanche about deciding such things. Interested readers, might be worth reading about a similar problem of neglect and laziness, that occurred in Chelsea and Westminster Hospital, during a night shift, where a paediatrician intentionally failed to do something to prevent a deteriorating baby from dying, because he wanted to spend private time with his girlfriend, the baby's nurse, who was on the same shift, and should have been looking after the baby, but left the ward to be with her Paediatrician boyfriend. Details of this case can be found at Twitter.com/TumTumTum.

♣ Who receives DNAR Orders?

Apparently, the elderly and mental health patients. Why? Perhaps it is because they are considered, by government, to be unproductive members of society, who use up valuable resources that the government would prefer to allocate to matters that reflect well on the government, and will help keep or gain new votes. Additionally, these patients are less likely to have the facility to vote in general elections, so they might be considered to have even less useful value.

♣ Cruelty and Power

Some people become doctors because of the power it gives them – the power of life and death. Such seemed to be the case with Harold Shipman, but his cannot have been a unique case. There are, indeed, many vicious and heartless doctors in the NHS, and working alongside these people is quite an education. Of course, it is not possible to forensically examine the conduct of such people – they make decisions that are rarely questioned, unless there is a good reason to investigate them, such as a larger than usual number of deaths of patients in their care. However, with a situation such as Covid-19, where killing off patients is not considered, by government, as a negative thing, then issuing DNARs can serve as a smokescreen for Harold Shipman type doctors who enjoy "allowing" patients to die.

♣ Summary

Issuing a DNAR order is an easy thing to do, is less work than treating the patient, poses no professional or criminal risk to the issuing doctor, permits racial or other types of discrimination, with respect to keeping patients alive or not, helps to improve a hospital's government imposed targets and, thereby, provides greater job security for the doctor and CEO, makes the government appear that they are doing a good job of managing the NHS, and direct resources in a way that is of benefit to them. DNARs are not patient centric!

5: AVOIDABLE PATIENT DEATHS

When a patient dies in hospital, due to mistakes by staff, the family of the deceased might expect that a legal Hearing will uncover issues of neglect or systemic failures. The following example of the British legal process might show how that expectation is an optimistic one.

The Incident

In 2015, Jacqueline Scott, 55, was an *Intensive Care* patient at St George's Hospital, Tooting. Jacqueline was unable to breathe for herself, so she was attached to a ventilator machine. During the night, the power supply to the ventilator failed, and the ventilator's backup battery power supply automatically took over, and the machine's audio-visual alarm system automatically activated.

Two of the shift nurses were alerted to the alarms, but they did not understand the flashing "battery" graphical symbols, so they ignored the alarms, in the hope that the problem would just go away.

Once the battery power had been drained, the ventilator stopped, and Jacqueline's normal breathing processes of gas exchange stopped. A few minutes later, Jacqueline died.

By ignoring the alarms, and not escalating the problem to more competent staff, such as an anaesthetist or a properly competent ICU nurse, the two nurses hoped to avoid drawing attention to their lack of competency, which is not too surprising, because they come from a part of the world that is well known for the ease at which nursing qualifications can be fraudulently obtained. Such incompetency is what makes staff, such as these, loyal to the NHS cover-up culture, because they rely on it to keep their jobs and registrations.

⚲ *The Royal Courts of Justice*

At the Coroner's Hearing, an expert witness, Dr Renate Wendler, Consultant Anaesthetist, offered several comments and opinions:

❶ She found evidence of good nursing practice and care.

❷ "Nurses were busy looking after Jacqueline in all sorts of ways."

❸ "The best nurses were looking after Jacqueline, but that they reviewed the design of the machine and felt it was not intuitive."

❹ "The ventilator made a loud screeching alarm that no nurse had previously heard. This noise must have been the final battery warning. A lot of high priority alarms had sounded."

❺ "It was not realistic to expect nurses to know when power would have been interrupted to the plug sockets."

❻ "We looked at Mrs Scott's health and we found she was very sick and probably a pre-terminal patient when she came to the hospital."

❼ "The hospital has since ensured all nurses are given formal training on how to use the ventilator and the alarms which sound when its power supply is disrupted."

♀ *Critique*

① The priority for preserving life is maintaining patency of a patient's airway, breathing, and circulation. This is why Jacqueline was connected to a ventilator – she could not maintain her own breathing. Jacqueline was certainly not subject to "good practice and care", because the nurses made no attempts to preserve her life.

② To say that nurses were looking after Jacqueline in "all sorts of ways" is an attempt to deflect attention from the fact that they were not really looking after her at all, because they were not complying with their primary duty, to keep her alive.

③ To claim that Jacqueline was in the care of the "best nurses" is an absolute assertion, which suggests that they are the best nurses that can be found anywhere. If the best nurses do not understand their jobs, are unwilling to request help so that they may propagate problems that they do not understand, to more capable staff, and are relaxed about letting a patient die, then they are the antithesis of what any reasonable person would describe as the "best nurses".

The claim that the ventilator machine was not intuitive is like saying that a wall power socket is not intuitive. Ventilators are specifically designed to be easy to use and, as with any other type of machine which requires power, knowing how to switch it on and off is pretty much idiot proof. To say that the machine was not intuitive to those very nurses who are responsible for ensuring that it is working is not based on logical reasoning, it is waffling diversion from the nurses' lack of competency. If none of the nurses were familiar with the ventilator then, either they should have raised this as a safety issue, at the start of their shift, or they should have consulted with an anaesthetist about who to call, in case they encountered any problems. Not knowing how something works is not a problem, but not doing anything about it is very much a problem, because it demonstrates no respect or understanding for the legal duty to reduce risk. *For those readers who are not familiar with medical ventilator systems, not understanding a power failure alarm is like a bus driver not knowing what a hand-brake is.*

④ The assertion that no nurse had previously heard the alarm is another absolute statement, meant to give the impression that alarms are never triggered, but that is a lie. At the start of any shift, it is the responsibility of all qualified staff to conduct machine checking protocols for ventilator and other machines, and this includes checking that the power disconnection alarms work. This is a simple thing to do, emergency nurses, paramedics, and anaesthetic technicians do it every day; it only requires switching the power to the machine off, ensuring that both audio and visual alarms are automatically activated, then switching the power back on, and ensuring that the resumption power silences the alarms.

⑤ The statement "It was not realistic to expect nurses to know when power had been interrupted" is absolutely right, that is why ventilators have power disconnection alarms to alert staff to the fact. What makes this statement such an obvious deception is the fact that the nurses did know that the power had been "interrupted", because the ventilator alarm drew their attention to the machine.

⑥ "Mrs Scott was probably pre-terminal" infers that she was going to die anyway, so the hospital's failure to keep her alive has no relevance. Yes, she was going to die – everybody does, but the hospital's duty is to preserve, improve, and extend life. Is the expert witness (anaesthetist) trying to suggest that Mrs Scott's care was palliative only? If so, that is something that would have been mentioned at the Hearing, but it wasn't mentioned, so it appears that this statement may be what is being described by the research performed by the *Dr Foster Intelligence* organisation, as detailed in the above sub-section "Hospitals Fiddling Death Rates".

⑦ "The hospital has since ensured that nurses are given training on how to use the ventilators." What? The nurses were given equipment training after a patient died, rather than before they started to become responsible for patient safety? This is outrageous stuff!

⑧ Every qualified and professionally registered clinical worker, such as a paramedic, nurse, or anaesthetic technician must, as part of their employment, undergo mandatory training and assessment of their life support skills. Foremost amongst these skills is the management of a patient's airway and breathing, including the use of a bag-valve-mask device, which is a manually operated ventilator that does not require a power supply, or any special skill to use it. A bag-valve-mask is stored with every ventilator, and is used when the ventilator fails, for whatever reason. In this case, when the ventilator finally stopped, the nurses should have called for help, and taken over the breathing task for Jacqueline, by using the bag-valve-mask device. The nurses did not do this, they failed their professional and registration duties, and so are a risk to patients. **The are fake nurses**.

⑨ The Coroner's Hearing did not raise the issue of the qualifications and competence of the nurses in whose care Jacqueline Scott was placed. Appropriate questions should have included: where did the nurses receive their training; what assessment methods did they have to pass before being allowed to register with the Nursing and Midwifery Council; were they assessed at all; who is responsible for ensuring that nurses meet proper safety criteria?

⑩ One other very significant factor that should be considered, about the Coroner's Hearing, is in regard to the expert witness, Dr Wendler. Did the Coroner know that she is employed by St George's Hospital? If so, why was she deemed to be an impartial expert witness?

According to the United Kingdom's *Crown Prosecution Service*:

> The duty of an expert witness is to help the court to achieve the objective by giving opinion which is **unbiased**, in relation to matters within their expertise. This is a duty that is owed to the court and overrides any obligation to the party from whom the expert is receiving instructions (Criminal Procedure Rule 19).
>
> Criminal Procedure Rule 19 obliges experts to disclose to the party instructing them anything of which the expert is aware that might reasonably be thought capable of undermining the expert's opinion, or detracting from their credibility or **impartiality**.

The CPS also stipulates disclosure of a conflict of interest of any kind, other than a potential conflict disclosed in the experts report.

Readers can decide for themselves whether or not the expert witness, in this case, had a conflict of interest.

⚱ *Reverse Logic*

Shortly after Jacqueline died, one of the anaesthetists asked the two nurses what they thought the reason was that her ventilator stopped working. The answer: "We thought it stopped because the patient died". The nurses thought that, instead of the ventilator keeping the patient alive, it was the patient that kept the ventilator functioning – the exact opposite of reality.

⚱ *Verdict*

As a result of the testimony from the expert witness, the cause of Jacqueline's death was deemed to be due to natural causes, neither the nurses nor the hospital itself were found culpable – in any way – and Jacqueline's family did not receive compensation for the failures of St George's Hospital.

⚰ **Baby Hayden**

Another example of an avoidable death, that is worth analysis, because it involved the worst kind of neglect, is that of six day old baby Hayden Ng, at a London Hospital.

Hayden's parents noticed that Hayden was becoming unresponsive, and was showing signs of distress, so they took him to Chelsea & Westminster Hospital, late one night (9 pm). A junior Doctor decided Hayden was ill enough to be admitted, and notified the night shift Consultant paediatrician. Immediately after starting his shift, the Consultant should have investigated his patients, including Hayden, and taken whatever steps were necessary to find the cause of Hayden's distress and breathing difficulties, and then prescribed a regime of treatments to reverse his deteriorating condition. However, the Consultant's girlfriend, a paediatric nurse, was also on the night shift, and so the Consultant decided to spend the vast majority of the shift alone, with her, in his office (door locked). Hayden's parents, however, were at his bedside throughout the night, and they could see that Hayden needed urgent attention, but their pleas to the nursing staff and paediatric doctors to do something to help Hayden were ignored.

During the night, and as part of his diagnostic regime, Hayden was subject to regular blood tests, known as Arterial Blood Gas reports, which showed that he was admitted with Type II severe respiratory failure, with both metabolic and respiratory acidosis, a condition that deteriorated from the time of admission, to the time of his death, eight hours later.

At the subsequent inquest, two expert witnesses, both Consultant anaesthetists, attested to the neglect, lack of care, and unprofessionalism of the Consultant paediatrician, and of the junior doctors who were also involved in Hayden's case. The experts stated that Hayden's death was avoidable, if he had received even the most basic of care. The experts also criticised the reluctance of all concerned to call for help from the on duty anaesthetists, who are the experts in dealing with respiratory failure, and who have well established protocols for reversing such conditions.

If, as the expert witnesses say, Hayden's death was avoidable, why did the paediatrician not take an interest in treating Hayden? The answer to that question lies in the fact that he spent the shift with his girlfriend, Hayden's nurse who, herself, neglected her duties, by abandoning Hayden to be with her boyfriend.

At the inquest, the paediatrician was ably defended by his brother, a barrister and Queen's Counsel. Hayden's parents could not afford such illustrious legal advocacy, and so their claim for negligence was dismissed, and the paediatrician avoided sanction.

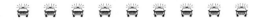

6: NHS PROPAGANDA

P ropaganda, which is the dissemination of information that is intended to influence a target audience, is one of the three factors that allow the NHS cover-up culture to be realised. Without propaganda, the NHS would not be able to so effectively deflect attention away from those matters that they prefer to hide from the public, so it is a subject that is of great importance to those officials who benefit from NHS "good news". {*The rules of propaganda are presented in Appendix 3*} Examples of propaganda include:

NHS Principles and Values

One of the ways that the NHS promotes itself is by use of seven *guiding NHS principles* and six *core values*. The *principles* describe the mission statement of the NHS, and includes such aims as "Working together for patients", and "Commitment to quality of care". The *core values* are very similar, and describe how the NHS intends to satisfy its stated principles with, for example, ensuring "quality of care", and "improving lives".

There is no auditing system to measure how the NHS meets its principles and values, and there is no punishment system for anyone who fails to comply with those principles and values. The reason being that the real purpose of the NHS principles and values is propaganda to appeal to the emotions of the public, by making them feel that they are safe in the care of the NHS.

Equal Opportunity Employer

By making the false claim that it provides equal opportunities for employees, the NHS is inferring that it is going above what is mandated, with respect to equality, making it a noble and meritocratic institution.

The claim that the NHS is an equal opportunity employer appeals to the emotions, and is a claimed policy that is in agreement with legislation (Equalities Act) – it cannot make a claim to the contrary, so the claim is redundant. By claiming that there is equality amongst employees, the NHS is inferring that equality (of treatment) extends to patients, which it does not, particularly with respect to older patients, who are often considered an annoyance and a threat to meeting "targets".

NHS and Hospital Policies.

All NHS work places use public relations style posters and intranet web pages to promote such drivers of professionalism as service quality and equality, honesty and openness, and freedom to raise issues (whistleblowing). These are *Ministry of Truth* style gimmicks which feed the public perception of the NHS satisfying its own constitutional principles and core values, whilst simultaneously appealing to public expectations of staff treatment, and quality of service delivery.

🚑 Duty of Candour

To make the public think that they have outlawed the practice of covering up medical errors, the government introduced, in 2014, Regulation 20 of the *Health and Social Care Act 2008 (Regulated Activities) Regulations*, which requires that the NHS admit to any mistakes made, and apologise to patients and their families for those mistakes. Regulation 20 is part of the NHS scheme for *Duty of Candour*. With this regulation, the public are meant to feel that they have the support of the government, should they fall victim to poor treatment and harm. Failure to comply with the duty of candour is a criminal offence, and victims are advised, in the first instance, to report failures to the Care Quality Commission who, surprisingly, have no power to investigate duty of candour matters, unless there is a serious contravention, which means patients have died. Reporting the CQC is very much a waste of time, and advice to contact them has the apparent intention of making it appear that the reported concerns will be properly addressed.

But, why would a hospital not comply with their duty of candour, and admit to their mistakes? The answer is that, by admitting to a mistake, it would trigger adverse press coverage against the hospital. Admission of culpability would also open up the path to negligence claims, and they would be accompanied by financial penalties, imposed by the courts. The hospital might also suffer an increase in indemnity insurance premiums. Significantly, a failure to comply with the duty of candour has never resulted in any individual suffering legal sanction; it is a law without teeth.

Duty of candour is, in effect, an implementation of the propaganda rule to "Evoke predictable responses in the target", with the aim of making the public feel that they can trust in the honesty of the NHS.

⛨ Hospital Values

In addition to the more general NHS values and principles, individual hospitals define their own values, usually four or five easy to remember concepts, which are known as "Trust Values", and use these as propaganda for public consumption.

Examples of hospital values are**: Teamwork, Respect, Intelligence, Professionalism,** and **Excellence.** Some hospital Trusts create "Trust Values" with catchy acronyms; the above values, for example, would have the acronym of TRIPE.

(Use of these values meets the goal of propaganda rule 12 – *Create a simple mantra*, with the view to satisfying propaganda rule 4: *Claim the same beliefs as the target.*)

Evidence that these hospital values are "spin", aimed at the public, lies in the fact that their use, as mantras, is duplicated throughout all public relations documents, and is usually displayed, as posters, in public areas of hospitals, often in main entrance thoroughfares. This is the NHS version of **"Arbeit macht frei!"**

⛨ Hospital Whistleblowing Policy

As a demonstration of a hospital's legally required support and encouragement for employees to speak out and raise concerns, the hospital will have a section of their employee intranet and publically accessible web sites dedicated to describing the rights and expectations of whistleblowers, and instructions as to how they should report their concerns. By doing so, the hospital hopes to provide "proof" that its beliefs, concerning raising of issues, intersect with the belief of the public, that whistleblowing is good for patient safety, and is encouraged.

This pro whistleblowing message is propaganda to convince the public that the NHS views on openness about patient safety are, indeed, correct and proper. Additionally, these official hospital statements of support, for the legal requirements to act in the public interest, help make the public feel that their NHS will always act in a way which produces the best outcome for them, and their families.

◢ Television Programmes

A contemporary example of how the NHS uses propaganda, disguised as public information, are the behind the scenes television programmes about the operational details of hospital accident and emergency departments. The message, in ALL episodes, is very positive and caring, and shows how staff treat each other with the same degree of dignity and respect that patients receive, and everyone is happy and respectful. Anyone watching these programmes will be so impressed with the effectiveness of care, and the 100% positive patient outcomes, that their contented emotions will migrate to all other aspects of the NHS, and they will feel that the NHS is safe in the current government's capable hands.

This type of public relations exercise is intended to portray the good works of A&E staff, but the public already have respect for the people who work in A&E, so the programme just repeats what we already know. The desired message is that hospital management and the Government, by association, are also acting in our best interests, so we should trust and support them, in turn. {*A propaganda analysis of television programmes features in Appendix 4}*

☁ Posters and Intranets

Part of a hospital's public relations (propaganda) strategy is to divert tax payer's money from its intended destination, which is clinical care, towards the generation of monthly magazine and web based staff support and clinical standards documents. Significant sections of these "spin" documents are devoted to positive stories of how patients have benefitted from treatment at the hospital, along with happy smiling group photographs of the patients, nursing staff, and managers. The intended effect of these positive public relations messages is to compensate for the absence of negative information concerning the experiences of those patients who have have poor experiences of NHS treatment. Without these positive propaganda broadcasts, their would be too much of an information void for the public to believe the NHS is performing as they would expect. In effect, NHS propaganda supports NHS cover-ups.

☁ Clinical Targets

One of the most significant vote losers for any government concerns patient waiting times, both for diagnostic and treatment services. To satisfy the demands of voters, targets for waiting times are used as devices to prove how well any component of the NHS is doing. If a patient does not receive their particular service within target guidelines, that will be a vote loser for the sitting government and, if that patient suffers as a consequence of delays, the case might be reported in the press, and that will become an impetus for voters to lose affiliation with the political party in power – another vote loser.

By broadcasting their successful meeting of clinical targets, the government complies with the propaganda rule to "create" the fact that targets are being met, by repeatedly claiming so. In the interest of balance, the NHS does have a lot of success in meeting targets, but the fact that the focus is on metrics, rather than quality of clinical outcomes is, itself, an aspect of propaganda, it deflects attention away from other issues, such as clinical mistakes, sepsis, and fraud.

✍ Single-use Blood Pressure Cuffs

A significant factor in patient deaths is that of cross contamination and infection, and one of the ways in which the NHS attempts to reduce person-to-person caused infections is by using single-use devices, such as blood pressure cuffs. This approach was introduced in the early part of the 21st century, as a reaction to the well publicised deaths due to hospital acquired (nosocomial) infections. Prior to the introduction of single-use blood pressure cuffs, it was normal for a cuff to be shared between patients, and cleaned with an appropriate disinfecting solution, after each patient had finished with it. With a single-use cuff, it is discarded immediately after use, thereby removing the possibility of cross infection which would otherwise occur with multi-use cuffs.

The problem is that the NHS does not supply enough blood pressure cuffs to allow single-patient use, so the single-use cuffs are reused, in exactly the same way that the multi-patient cuffs are reused. The NHS, of course, can quite reasonably declare that they supply single-use devices, even though these devices are reused between patients. What is really happening is implementation of rules of propaganda, specifically:

🕸 5 - Appeal to the target's emotions.

🕸 7 - Be selective with information.

🪰 Breathing Circuits

When a patient has a general anaesthetic, they need assistance with their breathing, and are supplied with oxygen and other breathing gases by means of a flexible breathing circuit, which is connected to an anaesthetic machine, controlled by an anaesthetist. If a breathing circuit is reused by other patients, it will pose a cross infection risk to those patients, by the possibility of passing, for example, Creutzfeldt–Jakob Disease (CJD), and blood borne viruses, such as human immunodeficiency virus (HIV) and Hepatitis.

To reduce the risk of cross contamination, the NHS uses single-use breathing circuits. However, just as with the issue of cost saving by reusing single-use blood pressure cuffs, breathing circuits are reused between patients, and are only routinely discarded on a weekly basis. As a workaround to using the same circuit for multiple patients, NHS hospitals stipulate that a single-use anti-bacterial/viral filter is placed between the patient and the breathing circuit. The problem is that there is no formal system of checks to ensure that someone has remembered to fit a new filter for each patient and, without a system that can catch instances of human error, the possibility of a filter being reused is a real one. The lesson that the NHS does not understand is that if failures can happen – then failures will happen, and this is an issue that is highly relevant for the contemporary problem of recurring coronavirus epi/pandemics.

Interested readers, who might want more details of this issue, can refer to various reports on the internet; for example:

https://www.birmingham.ac.uk/Documents/college-mds/haps/projects/cfhep/psrp/finalreports/PS022FinalReportDingwall.pdf

⛴ 7: PATIENT SAFETY

P atient safety is a key ingredient of a recipe for successful delivery of clinical services. Intuitively, then, it would seem to follow that the NHS must be immersed within a safety culture. It is not. The application of safety, particularly with respect to compliance with the *Health And Safety At Work Act*, is based on minimal compliance, professional requirements, and regulatory body guidelines and codes of practice. These external impositions do successfully (in the main) deliver safety, primarily because they are the easiest things to do, but these impositions can be regarded more as mandatory and minimum ways of service delivery, or even as safety nets to catch hazards, rather than meeting the terms of a safe working environment. Compliance with these regulatory requirements does not make a safety culture; it makes a compliance culture - there is a difference. When someone works in a way which is compliant with established requirements, it means doing something in a particular way because they have to; they are ticking the boxes. Conversely, when performing a task in a way which is not standard, but is the safest method, then that can be considered to be complying with the attributes of a safety culture. It is the outcome which is of importance – not the method, and not just ticking the right boxes.

✍ NHS Attitude To Safety

In the NHS, safety is achieved in a manner which is based on minimality (only do what is mandated), and is subordinate to the management imperative of meeting government targets. One sign that those significant components of the NHS - hospitals - do not accept safety as being a driver of behaviours, lies in the fact that their Boards of Directors do not include dedicated and properly qualified Safety Directors but, instead, they appoint non-executive Directors, or Directors of Nursing, but without giving them the executive power to ensure safety. Such an appointment serves to give the impression that safety is taken seriously, but this, once again, is just a public relations tactic, for the benefit of the public.

A truer reflection of patient safety lies in the figures. For example, the *Summary Hospital-level Mortality Indicator* has shown that there may be as many as one hundred unnecessary patient deaths a day, in England and Wales. The unnecessary death rates are so disproportionately high, that the Department of Health has instructed hospitals to publish their annual figures for patient deaths, presumably to embarrass them into correcting the problems which cause the deaths. It can be argued that, because they did not previously publish these figures, voluntarily, then hospitals have been covering up the figures for patient deaths and, given that the Department of Health acknowledges that the NHS has a cover-up culture, it seems reasonable to make such an assertion. (Reducing the number of unnecessary deaths is not the same as recording a reduced number of deaths in official documents – fiddling the figures is part of the "cover-up" process)

▪ Safety Culture

> The safety culture of an organisation is the product of individual and group values, attitudes, perceptions, competencies, and patterns of behaviour that determine the commitment to, and the style and proficiency of an organisation's health and safety management. Organisations with a positive safety culture are characterised by communications founded on mutual trust, by shared perceptions of the importance of safety, and by confidence in the efficacy of preventive measures. (*Health and Safety Executive, 1993*).

For an NHS safety culture to exist, all staff must comply with the above characteristics of a safety culture, described thus:

▪ Individual Values

If all NHS employees possessed the values that support a safety culture, then they would all feel free to exercise their right to blow the whistle about whatever safety or other issue they may have identified. If that were the case, the NHS would be regarded as an open honest environment in which to work, and there would not be any negative press about the NHS being a bullying and "cover-up" organisation. As this is not the case then, by inference, the lack of individual values is evidence that the NHS does not have a safety culture.

▪ Group Values

For particular staff groups, such as those of a particular hospital ward, to possess equally shared values concerning safety, the members of the group would have to consider themselves to be equal, both as employees and human beings, and there would not be any compromising of the attributes for a meritocratic and equal society. There would not exist, for example, divisions based on personal or professional jealousies, favouritism, or discrimination. Favouritism and discrimination are part of the culture of the NHS, and this fact gives more evidence that the absence of group values means that the NHS does not respect the culture of safety.

📇 Attitudes

The commitment to a safety culture is dependent on NHS employees and managers having a comprehensive understanding of factors which degrade safety, and the legal requirements for identifying hazards, measuring risk, and creating systems of work, and their associated staff training, which meet the legally binding imperative to reduce risk to as low as reasonably practicable. The NHS attitude to safety revolves around the principle of how best to cover up safety issues, and this is evidence, once again, that NHS attitudes to safety run contrary to a positive safety culture.

📇 Competencies

Professional competencies are dependent on employees possessing the appropriate level of intelligence and training which their particular roles and registration requirements demand. The NHS employs many clinical professionals who are fraudulently qualified and incompetent (discussed later) but, because they are loyal to their employer's cover-up culture, their positions remain secure. Again, the absence of an NHS safety culture is evidenced by the NHS practice of employing people who are fraudulently "qualified" for their roles.

◪ Patient Abuse

An issue that NEVER receives public recognition, but deserves mention, is that of hostility that many clinical staff, particularly nurses and HCAs (Health Care Assistants), have towards patients, which can can be illustrated by the growing practice of foreign nurses "talking over" patients in their own languages, particularly when their team leaders or managers (matrons) are also foreign. This is a particular problem with East European, Spanish, South African, and Filipino nurses, who will chatter away, pretending to not recognise the English language, and completely ignore requests for information or help from patients who might, for example, need to visit the toilet, or are developing pressure sores, and so on. Even without proof from audio recordings, the way these staff laugh and joke, as they walk away from the patient needing help, is very obvious. Of course, it is not just foreign staff who are guilty of abusing patients, some British staff, particularly (for some reason) HCAs are also hostile, but more in their negative actions and inactions, rather than in speech, although this "rule" is ignored for elderly patients – perhaps because staff think that all elderly patients are senile, and incapable of reporting the abuse they experience.

◪ Patterns of Behaviour

Satisfying the above issues is the test which helps determine whether or not an organisational safety culture exists. In all cases, the test fails. Attitudes are based on self preservation; if, for example, an employee can be held accountable for failing to meet a government target, the employee, whose position is at risk, because of the failure to meet the said target, will use whatever cover-up culture tricks, such as blame passing, to protect their position.

"**Organisations with a positive safety culture are characterised by communications founded on mutual trust, by shared perceptions of the importance of safety, and by confidence in the efficacy of preventive measures.**" *Health and Safety Executive, 2019.*

Shared Safety Perceptions

If all components of the NHS perceived the issue of safety in the same way, there would not be any need for anyone to blow the whistle. In the NHS, there is no shared perception of safety.

Confidence in Preventive Measures

If NHS (particularly hospital) managers and directors had confidence in their safety related preventative measures, realising those preventative measures would have to be standard practice, and that would entail compliance with the *Precautionary Principle* (described in Appendix 6), but this is something which nobody in the NHS ever mentions, or takes action on.

If the NHS had a safety culture, it would satisfy all of the above components of such a culture, including compliance with both the Precautionary Principle, and the Health and Safety at Work Act duty to reduce risk to as low as reasonably practicable. That would be the foundation on which the safety culture is built, and there would be no need for a cover-up culture to exist. Indeed, a cover-up culture, by its definition, cannot coexist with a safety culture. An NHS cover-up culture, however, does exist, and its existence has been identified and accepted as being real, by the government. Again, it follows, then, that the NHS does not have a safety culture.

◉ British Social Attitudes Survey (2014)

To put the above discourse into a social context, the King's Fund have produced the following results of the British Social Attitudes survey into the public response to the question "How much do you trust NHS nurses, doctors, and managers to put the interests of patients above the interests of the hospital and staff?". For **nurses** the answer was 21%. Trust in **doctors** was 17%. For **managers**, the figure was only 2.5%. Perhaps there is wisdom in crowds.

◉ Safety versus Cover-ups

There is a conflict between the desire, by the public (service users), for the NHS to have an ingrained safety culture, and the incentives of NHS officials (service providers) to conceal, disguise, and deny instances of poor care, particularly avoidable patient deaths. What the public want is for the NHS to comply with its founding principles, as mandated in the *NHS Constitution*, which is to **work at the limits of science to save lives and improve physical and mental health and wellbeing**. To meet these constitutional requirements, the NHS would have to be a meritocratic employer, where staff are treated fairly and equally, are properly remunerated for their labours; are proven, by independent bodies, to be properly competent and qualified, can safely associate, communicate, and cooperate with service providers and users alike, and are disbarred for being drug users or any other reasons where they increase risk. In complying with the goal of saving and improving lives, NHS staff would feel free to meet the requirement to be open and candid about mistakes and failures – without fear of retribution.

By being open about failures, rather than covering them up, regarding failures and mistakes, the rest of the NHS would learn from those failures and, by so doing, the learning experience will reduce the likelihood of clinicians repeating well known mistakes.

For hospital Chief Executives, and other NHS officials, the above description of a meritocratic and honest work environment would mean that details of incidents of avoidable harm would enter the public domain, and that would reflect badly on those officials and the government alike. For hospital Chief Executives, their job security and lucrative pay, benefits, and pension schemes could be compromised by the resultant bad publicity whereas, if no such adverse publicity occurred, their suitability for their jobs would not come under scrutiny; as of 2020, the average salary for a Chief Executive is approximately £280,000 per annum. However, the overall package, including pensions, freebies, and taxable benefits that they do NOT pay tax on, takes the overall sum to nearer £500,000 per annum.

So, the motivation for Chief Executives to protect their lucrative positions is clear – money! With that aim in mind, Chief Executives "dissuade" employees from raising concerns about issues that would reflect badly on them – hence the NHS cover-up culture.

* * *

A secretive and poorly understood reason why Chief Executives are not deterred from establishing cover-up practices, is because the NHS Confederation requires that Chief Executives ensure that positive reputations are established for their clinical establishments, under the guidance of "Reputation Management" lawyers.

This conflict between a culture of safety, and a culture of cover-ups, can be exemplified by the Royal Shrewbury & Telford Hospital's Maternity Unit scandal, where as many as 1,200 deaths of babies may have been due to sub-standard care, and dating as far back as the 1960's. During the investigation – 2017 onwards - by Donna Ockenden (midwife), the Chief Executive informed her that the failings at his hospital Trust were false, and the negative media reports were scaremongering because they, the media, especially the BBC, "had it in for him". This attitude was raised by a House of Commons statement by Lucy Allan, MP, who stated "The question we have to keep asking is whether the denial and normalisation of poor care is a systemic problem within the complex bureaucracy that is the NHS". There lies the true state of NHS attitudes towards patient safety; denying that medical failures occur is normal practice, and is part of the unwritten ethos of NHS management.

Note: A list of factors that increase risk can be found in Appendix 10.

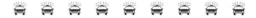

⛑ 8: INFORMED CONSENT

A s part of the safety protocol for patients undergoing NHS care, it is essential that those patients are given the opportunity to discuss, understand, and agree with the course of actions that are proposed for them by Doctors (surgeons, anaesthetists) giving that care, so that Doctors can gain *Informed Consent* from patients, to proceed with their treatment.

For minor matters, such as taking blood pressure, consent can be verbal, or it can be implied, such as when the patient raises their arm to accept the blood pressure cuff. For more in-depth treatment, such as anaesthetic and surgical processes, the patient must give written (signed) consent, after being informed, by the doctor doing the treatment, of the details of that treatment, the alternatives, and the benefits and risks of each available option.

Informed Consent documents differ between hospitals, but the principles for Consent are standardised by the General Medical Council (GMC), some of which are listed in Appendix 11.

When a particular course of treatment turns out as expected, the Informed Consent process appears to have achieved its purpose but, if there is an adverse outcome, or the patient's treatment does not match what was consented to, the Consent form might be retrospectively altered, or "lost", so that the doctor concerned can protect themselves from culpability, by altering what the patient consented to. In these cases, the Informed Consent process is revealed for what it really is, which is a means by which the hospital or doctor can defend themselves, in court, by claiming that treatment matched what was written in the Consent form, or that the patient cannot complain about the treatment they received, because they were informed of the risks etc, and agreed to accept those risks.

⚔ Relevant GMC Informed Consent Guidelines

♟ The doctor and patient make an assessment of the patient's condition, taking into account the patient's medical history.

♟ In assessing the risk to an individual patient, you (Doctor) must consider the nature of the patient's condition, their general health and other circumstances. These are variable.

♟ You must tell the patient if an investigation or treatment might result in an adverse outcome, even if the likelihood is very small.

♟ You (doctor) must provide the patient with information about the potential benefits, risks and burdens, and the likelihood of success, for each option; this should include information, if available, about whether the benefits or risks are affected by which organisation or doctor is chosen to provide care.

♟ You must use the patient's medical records or a consent form to record the key elements of your discussion with the patient.

♟ Involve other members of the healthcare team in discussions with the patient.

♟ In order to have effective discussions with the patient about risk, you must identify the adverse outcomes that may result from the proposed options. This includes the potential outcome of taking no action. Risks can take a number of forms, but will usually be:

☞ Side effects

☞ Complications

☞ Failure of an intervention to achieve the desired aim.

❧ Give the patient the information they need in a way they can understand.

❧ Ensure the patient understands the given information.

❧ The patient has a right to seek a second opinion.

❧ Give the patient time to reflect, before and after they make a decision, especially if the information is complex, or what you are proposing involves significant risks.

* * *

To understand why the Consent process is corrupt, it is useful to analyse the above GMC mandated procedural points, and illustrate failure of the process, using the case of a patient, Dinara Farina.

🚑 Dinara Farina

In her book, *Stabbed in the Back,* Dinara describes her childbirth experience in a West London hospital, where none of the midwives or doctors (obstetricians or anaesthetists) considered how her previous pelvic injury from a car crash would prevent her from having a natural birth delivery, due to her inability to "dilate" sufficiently. By treating Dinara as just another patient on the deliveries board, doctors failed to treat her as an individual, and consider her particular medical history (pelvic injury), so they made her suffer past her normal delivery date, and wasted time in persistently injecting her with drugs to "induce" her to deliver, for a dangerously long time after her waters broke, which put her unborn baby at severe risk of infection. All this time, of course, Dinara was experiencing increasing levels of pain. It was only after maternity staff started to become irritated by Dinara's failure to deliver, and the consequent degradation to the Obstetric department target to minimise the time before patients are discharged, that staff responded to Dinara's requests for help that an anaesthetist recommended pain relief via epidural anaesthesia, which required Dinara's Informed Consent – she was given a BLANK Consent Form to sign. An hour after giving Dinara the epidural, the anaesthetist visited her to check the effectiveness of the epidural, and found it was not working, because he had put it in the wrong place, leaving her with permanent injury. After a wait of another 3 hours, the anaesthetist removed the epidural catheter from Dinara's back.

☠ Informed Consent Failures

The anaesthetist conducted the Informed Consent process in a way that did not correctly comply with professional requirements, as detailed in Appendix 11:

🕸 He explained the risks of epidural block, but did not mention "adhesive arachnoiditis", which is where the anaesthetist accidentally inserts a needle too far into the back, pierces the dura membrane, injects into the arachnoid space, and causes adhesion of nerve bundles, causing a life long and severely painful condition.

🕸 Dinara's failure to "dilate", and her prolonged time past delivery date, did not prompt investigation by midwives or doctors, and there was no attempt to consider how her previous pelvic injury was the cause of her inability to deliver naturally.

🕷 At no stage was Dinara informed that she could request an independent second medical opinion.

🕷 By giving written consent to an epidural, immediately before being given the epidural, Dinara did not have the time to research or consider the implications or alternatives to the epidural.

🕷 When the anaesthetist went through the Consent process with Dinara, she was in distress, and in great pain, so she was not in a condition to think about what she was being told about the epidural risks and alternatives, so she just went along with what the anaesthetist told her, trusting him, and was led, by him, to the decision that HE preferred, which was to have the epidural block.

🕷 At no stage did anybody inform Dinara of how the epidural block success rate at the hospital compare with other hospitals.

🕷 When the anaesthetist inserted the epidural, it went into Dinara's middle back (T6), rather than the usual place, which is the lower back (L3), but the anaesthetist fraudulently recorded, in the **blank** Consent form that Dinara signed, that he placed the epidural at L3.

* * *

Fortunately, Dinara delivered a healthy baby, by caesarian section but, unfortunately, Dinara's epidural injection had caused her to suffer adhesive archnoiditis, and she subsequently spent several years in great pain. Adhesive arachnoiditis is so rarely known by Doctors of all types, that it is usually confused with fibromyalgia and post-natal psychological changes, so it was only by accident that she eventually discovered the truth about what happened to her, and the mistake that her anaesthetist made in her epidural.

In her research into adhesive arachnoiditis, Dinara triggered an investigation by the hospital, and that investigation resulted in the denial that her condition was caused by a faulty epidural block. The report also made the blatant lie that the anaesthetist who gave her the epidural had left the hospital, and his whereabouts were unknown when, in fact, he was still working at the hospital. Indeed, quite shockingly, Dinara discovered that the person who conducted the investigation was none other than the consultant anaesthetist who gave her adhesive arachnoiditis injury.

* * *

Clearly, the Informed Consent process does not guarantee that the patient is fully informed of the risks of, and alternatives to, their care. Neither does written Consent guarantee that the care they receive matches what is recorded on the Consent form. Most noteworthy is the way in which a patient's signature is regarded as "proof" that they accept, understand, and are aware of all of the risks they face, even though the patient could only understand those things if they, themselves, were qualified medical doctors.

As a mark of how corrupt a doctor can be, Dinara's anaesthetist made her sign a blank Consent form, so that he could cover himself, should he make a mistake, by retrospectively entering a warning about the particular mistake he made, and with Dinara's signature falsely confirming that she was warned about the particular problem, and accepted the accompanying risks.

☠ Tip For Surgical Patients

Immediately after signing your Consent form, photograph every page, and email the images to yourself. Then, if the Consent form is maliciously modified, lost, you lose your copy, or you lose your phone, you will still have a copy of the original form. This same rule applies to all documents, because they will be amended or destroyed, if that protects hospitals and clinicians.

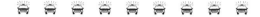

9: ROGUE CLINICAL WORKERS

There are approximately one million clinical professionals in the United Kingdom, including 500,000 nurses, and 300,000 doctors. The majority of these are conscientious and well meaning people, who take pride in their work, and who will always do what is best for patients. The importance of these people is directly reflected by their description as "key workers" and, without them, society would be uncompassionate, cruel, and characterised by *survival of the fittest*.

Unfortunately, alongside these valuable key workers, there is a significant minority who, to varying degrees, are: dishonest, antisocial, violent, sex predators, addicted to drugs, unreliable, unsafe, uncaring and, as is mentioned elsewhere in this text, fraudulently qualified for the posts they hold. The negative and dangerous effects of these "rogue" elements are disproportionately higher than their numbers represent, and they pose a constant risk to patients, with the risk they pose only moderated by the rescuing effects of their more competent and conscientious peers. The contribution that these rogues make to the health and welfare of patients is, at best, minimal and, at worst, deadly. For the NHS, the value of these people is limited to their loyalty to the cover-up culture, which they rely on, and in the making up of staff numbers – they help managers meet government directed staffing level targets.

Although these rogues may not have difficulty in bluffing their way through nursing and other training courses – that is very easy to do. However, their undesirable characteristics and behaviours does not mean that these rogue elements are effectively filtered out of the system; far from it, many of these people are promoted through the management hierarchy, and achieve a relatively higher degree of job success and security than their more able colleagues. The reason for their career success is because these are some of the most loyal sycophants to their immediate managers, and they can always be relied upon to support the cover-up culture that protects both themselves, and their managers (Chapter 13 repeats this point). It is only when their behaviour results in intolerable and publicised (cover-up failure) harm to patients, that these rogues are removed from their positions and, in some cases, also removed from their professional registers. The following examples provide a flavour of some of the types of people employed by the NHS:

"Rogue" Clinical Professionals

Dr Mohsan Answar, Anglesey

Police discovered he had extreme pictures of sexual abuse of a nine year old boy, and pictures of men having sex with animals. He pleaded ignorance, but the police found that he was a member of a WhatsApp group that shared images.

Nurse Imelda Azubuike (critical care), Glasgow

Miscalculated and administered ten times the prescribed dose of drug to one patient; increased another patient's drug infusion rate from 1 ml to 10 ml per hour; made several other medication errors; incapable of dispensing intravenous drugs (an easy task); printed a blood label for the wrong patient (deadly); ignored a patient's detached chest drain; miscellaneous other failures.

Note: Generally, critical care nurses have a well deserved reputation for their superior knowledge, education, and skills, but the NHS is renowned for its ineffective staff screening processes, and prioritising staffing level targets over safety.

♀ Nurse Subiah Kousar Akram, Huddersfield
Over two years, repeatedly accessed the medical records of a relative she did not like, and shared the information with people in her community.

♀ Nurse Violeta Aylward, Devizes
Accepted a shift in an Intensive Care Unit (ICU), without ICU experience, training, or qualifications; switched off a patient's ventilator, then attempted to switch it back on, but did not know how to do so. The patient needed emergency life support as a result.

♀ Dr Virginia Bodescu (paediatrician), Epsom
Two year suspension for having an unsafe level of English language ability. Parents reported that she did not understand patient notes, what parents told her about their childrens' conditions, so she did not understand what the health problems were. In an attempt to convince her Tribunal panel that she had excellent English language skills, she tried to convince them that she had worked as a teacher of English in Romania.

☠ Nurse Adrienn Bordas, Belfast

Failed to clean wounds properly. Failed to wash her hands after contact with a patients' wounds. Did not wear gloves. Lack of basic nursing skills. Lack of ability to communicate in English. Gave patients the wrong drugs. Gave false job references.

☠ Nurse Paul Bradford, Carstairs

Together with a health care assistant, Bradford encouraged one violent patient to punch another patient, who was autistic.

☠ Midwife Scott Butler, St George's Trust

Arrested at work for uploading over 400 images of paedophile rape, of children as young as four years, and people having sex with animals.

☠ Nurse Steven Campbell, Glasgow

Dragged an 88 year old dementia patient, with arthritis and a heart complaint, by her ankles, to her room. The event was witnessed by the patient's relatives.

☠ Paramedic Dominic Colella, London

After responding to an emergency call for a patient with a head injury, Colella stopped to have a haircut, whilst the patient was in the ambulance. He also interrupted transporting another patient (85 year old with severe blood poisoning) to hospital, to go shopping at Marks and Spencer.

☠ Nurse Karen Costello (care home), Chorley

Failed to administer blood thinning drugs, putting an elderly resident at risk of cardiac arrest. Failed to record drug stock levels. Neglected to record patient monitoring results.

☠ Nurse Philomena David, Kent

Gave an MMR jab to a 6 month old baby, when 12 months is the minimum age for jabs. Consistently failed to understand her job as a nurse. Could not work without supervision.

☠ Director of Nursing Hazel Dinnie, Aberdeen

Intimidated and threatened staff to deter them from reporting concerns and problems. Bullied staff into resigning.

☠ Senior Nurse Filomena Divinagracia, Glasgow

A nurse with ten years experience, only had the skills of a basic healthcare assistant. Had no knowledge of healthcare principles - not even the most basic skills of a qualified nurse. Could not work unsupervised. Had to be prompted to complete her duties.

☠ Nurse Francesco Gatta, Southend

A known risk to patients: could not speak English; connected a contaminated intravenous line to a patient; did not help a patient whose oxygen supply became detached, and was at risk of cardiac arrest; refused to attend a language assessment; incorrectly recorded a patient as being alert and breathing adequately; did not make regular blood pressure observations; put a sponge in a patient's mouth, and left it there.

☠ Paramedic Andrew Grant, Birmingham

Made indecent photos of children, and distributed them on the internet.

☠ Nurse David Hadfield, Blackburn

When attending to a confused 72 year old and terminally ill patient, who was very distressed, the nurse head-butted the patient – three times, causing cuts to the patient's forehead. He was sentenced to fifteen months in prison.

☠ Nurse Susan James, Salford

When in charge of a ward with 24 patients, 2 of whom where clinically unstable, she left 40 minutes early, claiming her car was broken. Consistently failed to maintain important clinical records.

☠ Dr Puja Kalia (trainee GP), Surrey

One year suspension by the Medical Practitioners Tribunal service for lying about passing exams, and creating forged qualification certificates to support her lies.

☠ Mental Health Nurse Mohamed Kamara, Bart's Trust

Raped a patient with post traumatic stress disorder and depression. He drew curtains around her bed, then tried to force sleeping pills into her mouth, before raping her. He was imprisoned for 15 yrs.

☠ Nurse Aaron Kibaja (ward manager), Nottinghamshire

Sexual harassment of female nurses, culminating in setting off a fire alarm, in a dementia ward, so that he could see a nurse's breasts bounce up and down. (The alarm could have triggered elderly and fragile patients to suffer cardiac arrest.)

☙ Nurse Lea Ledesma, Heart Hospital, London

When instructed to give a unit of blood to a patient who she had previously given a unit, she failed to validate the patient details (patient notes) with the label on the blood bag. She knew the patient's name, but saw that the name on the blood bag was for another patient. She then asked the patient his date of birth, and confirmed the date matched on the patient's wrist identity bracelet, rather than validating it against the date of birth on the blood bag label (soooo stupid) and patient notes. Even though she knew that the patient name on the blood bag label did not match the patient's name, she decided it must be the right blood, because she (incorrectly) confirmed that the date of birth was correct, so she gave the patient the blood, and he died several hours later. She was charged with manslaughter, but did not receive a fine or custodial sentence – only loss of registration. The sentencing Judge decided to give a light sentence, because Ledesma provided lots of very positive and supportive references from her colleagues (fellow countrymen). Curiously, neither the pathologist nor the coroner thought to test her English language skills, which were almost certainly a factor in her failures.

☙ Nurse Mun Lai Mah, Surrey

Gave a patient double the normal dose of insulin, without checking the patient's prescription chart, and failed to report or record giving the drug. Inserted the wrong size catheter.

☙ Dr Adrian Marsden (psychiatrist), Pebble Lodge, Poole

Discovered to have over 2,000 images of child sex abuse images on his computer and phone. He claimed that the pleasure he had from watching child abuse was his way of stress relief. Sentenced to an 18 month community service order.

♣ Nurse Juleth McKenzie, Bradford

With eight years post-qualifying experience, and a B.Sc. degree in Nursing, McKenzie did not understand the difference between micrograms and milligrams; could not calculate drug dosages; could not calculate heart rate, from a patient's pulse; gave a diabetic patient a drink of Lucozade, instead of the prescribed intravenous Glucose; was asked to check a patient's blood pressure, but checked the temperature instead.

♣ Nurse Fariba Mirtorabi, Margate

Neglected to administer blood thinning drug to patient at risk of pulmonary embolism and cardiac arrest. Recorded wrong dosages in a patient's records, administered four times the proper dose; going to sleep when she should have been tending to patients. Neglecting to record issuance of controlled drugs. Lied about her work experience.

♣ Nurse Tsvetanka Miteva, Rutland Care Village

After four years on the NMC register of nurses, she was so incompetent, dangerous, and unwilling to attend clinical and English language lessons, her employer reported her to the NMC for failures, including: Did not dispose of contaminated gloves in the clinical waste bin; Ignored patient's dangerously low blood pressure; Offered patient tea when she was losing consciousness; Was unable to state the normal values for oxygen saturation and respiration rate; Unable to take blood sugar readings; Attempted to apply a new dressing without firstly removing the dirty dressing; Copied what had been previously written in care and monitoring plans; Offered one colleague, who had collapsed, tea when other colleagues were trying to put her in the recovery position; Tried to check a patient's sacrum (lower back) whilst the patient was in the dining room; Placed Temazepam (psychoactive drug) in the cupboard of the wrong patient; Did not have the necessary knowledge of English to practise safely.

☠ Nurse Tamas Mocsari (care home), Reigate

Cannot communicate in English. Did not: report a fall by an elderly patient, record the patient's vital signs, check the patient for injury, create an incident form, initiate a risk assessment, update the patient's care plan. Removed another patient's catheter - without knowing how to do so, or recording the action in the care plan. Ignored the patient's claims of severe abdominal pain. Failed to call 999 when the patient needed emergency treatment.

☠ Nurse Mmpatji Motaung (care home), Bridgnorth

Assaulted an 80 year old dementia patient, at least three times. Allowed the same patient to fall on the floor, resulting in a fractured hip. Failed to check the patient for injuries, record the fall in the patient's notes, or inform other staff from next shift. Struck off and sentenced to six months in prison.

☠ Nurse Shiona Nelson, Kirkcaldy

Told a dying patient "It's time for the big sleep" in front of the patient's family. Told a student nurse to use the patient to practice taking blood samples on.

☠ Nurse Beaullah Ntsulumbana, Devon & Exeter Trust

When an elderly patient, distressed and suffering from a urinary infection, could not keep quiet, nurse Ntsulumbana taped his mouth shut, and told him, 3 times, that she was going to shoot him. The NMC gave her a caution.

☠ Nurse Bethany Oughton, Norfolk and Suffolk Trust

Police stopped her car, when she was on duty, on her way to a mental health patient, and found she was under the influence of cocaine. Although she was a danger to both road users and her patients, her Trust's Chief Nurse, Diane Hill, was satisfied that a 18 month driving ban was sufficient punishment, and neither the Trust or Nursing and Midwifery Council took further action against her. Some months later, Oughton was promoted (to band 7).

☠ Nurse Beverley Palmer, Southport

Failing to monitor a diabetic patient's blood sugar levels. Failed to administer insulin. Allowed the patient to deteriorate to point of diabetic coma, cardiac arrest, and near death (another nurse caught the problem just in time).

☠ Nurse Cristina Pereira, Norfolk & Norwich

Put patients at risk because she could not speak or read English; could not complete or patient records or comply with care plans; failed to give medication when it was needed, when was prompted to give medication she did not know how; refused to take an English test; refused to communicate with the NMC.

☠ Abdul Pirzada, Birmingham

A Pakistani, who claimed to be an asylum seeker from Afghanistan, used fake CV and qualifications, including a diploma for a medical degree, to gain work as a nurse and locum doctor at three Birmingham health centres - for seven years. His CV included claims to have worked as a doctor for the Red Cross and a Glasgow hospital, but nobody thought to check his claims. Pirzada prescribed incorrect drugs for patients (spotted by a pharmacist); stole drugs and prescription forms. Abdul Pirzada's real name is unknown, he assumed the name Abdul Pirzada - a famous Pakistani politician. "Pirzada" was sentenced to 18 months in prison, but allowed to keep his UK residency.

☠ Physiotherapist Adel Abdel Razeq, London

Whilst treating a patient, instructed her to remove her bra and underwear, inserted his fingers into her vagina, and asked if she used sex toys.

☠ Nurse Nuno Rodrigues (A & E), Plymouth

Sent explicit pictures of himself to a 13 year old girl.

☠ Nurse Proscovia Nakaggwa Sendjja, Whittington

Suspended for one year for discarding the care plan of a patient with a severe head injury, and replaced it with a fake care plan; recorded that the patient's condition as being less severe than previously recorded, and substantiated her fake diagnosis by forging a doctor's signature. The patient was subsequently diagnosed with a brain haemorrhage.

☠ Nurse James Snow (care home manager), Widnes

Persistent cruelty to patients, and falsifying treatment records. He repeatedly took food from patients; left a wheelchair bound patient in an isolated corridor, when other staff moved her back to the lounge, he would immediately move her back, to upset and frighten her.

☠ Paramedic Gabor Tekeres, Liverpool

Did not use safe patient handling techniques. Forced an 80 year old, who fell over, to stand up by herself, and did not make usual injury/health observations. Failed to inform the hospital that he was bringing a stroke victim. Drove his ambulance dangerously, without good reason. Was aggressive to patients. Inserted a cannula into a patient's vein without cleaning the skin first, without wearing gloves, and he put the cannula in his mouth. Did not know how to insert breathing tubes (endotracheal tube, laryngeal mask airway) when attending a heart attack victim, and did not give the patient oxygen; failed four mandatory trauma and life support and assessments.

☠ Nurse Jongo Vandi, Broadmoor

Started a fight with a psychiatric patient, and kicked him in the head – three times. He had to be pulled away by other staff.

☠ Nurse Grzegorz Wawrzynczak, Addenbrooke's Hospital

In the major trauma intensive care unit, assaulted and abused an elderly patient, causing physical and psychological harm.

☠ Neo-natal Nurse Craig Wilson, Glasgow

Failed to help a premature baby to breathe, by neglecting to switch on her humidifier. The baby died. His employer claimed that he was an ongoing risk to patients.

☠ Biomedical Scientist Jacqueline Wozniak, Buckinghamshire

On a number of occasions, recorded a false pathology test result but did not conduct the tests. Incorrectly interpreted test results for several patients.

☠ Nurse Uyabongeka Yengwa (nursing home), Cornwall

Nine month nursing suspension: Would not cooperate with British colleagues. Took a five hour sleep break on a night shift. Failed to monitor patients. Informed the wrong family after a patient died. Did not respond to an emergency call. Did not know the emergency services phone number (999).

☠ Biomedical Scientist Zhelana Atanasove, West Sussex

Failed to understand basic pathology identification techniques, or different media types, Did not inform microbiologists results of tests. Reported incorrect bacteriology results for several patients.

☠ Dr Asef Zafar, Surrey

For twelve years, whilst employed by the NHS, boosted his income by £350,000 per year, by authorising fraudulent personal injury claims.

🐞 Nursing and Midwifery Council

The failings of the NMC are discussed in several chapters, and it seems appropriate to repeat some of those failings here.

Note 1: The failure of the NMC to proactively protect the public, by neglecting to screen and effectively audit applicants for registration, is a failure that is duplicated by the Health and Care Professions Council (HCPC), who are the registration body for allied health professions.

Note 2: Ordinarily, when someone is critical of their registration body, they can expect imposition of the typical bullying response of the NHS cover-up culture, which is to suspend or remove their registration. It is only when their whistleblowing actions have resulted in career termination that whistleblowers feel free to exercise their rights of free speech, in revealing the truth about how these bodies fail the public.

British Trained Nurses

The purpose of a registration body (NMC, HCPC, GMC) is to protect the public from coming to harm from incompetent and dangerous individuals who adopt careers in healthcare professions, as exemplified by the above list of "rogues". To that aim, it would seem prudent that the registration bodies would ascertain the validity of an applicant for joining a professional register, but they do not do this. Instead, they entrust the veracity of the applicant's training institution, who inform the registration body of the applicant's successful completion of their training course, as proof that they are suitable to be accepted as a Registered Nurse, Paramedic etc.

A significant problem with allowing universities to attest to the suitability of their students to be enrolled on a professional register lies in the motivations of the universities. If a university has high standards for passing a nursing course, for example, there will be a relatively higher number of failures and, because of the high failure rate, the university may fail to attract enough students to fill all of their training places. Consequently, the university will also fail to receive as much funding that they would otherwise receive, if they had lower standards and a higher pass rate.

The extra funding due to a higher pass rate is what motivates the universities to push as many people through the training system as they can. The issue of the students being safe to work as healthcare professionals is something that universities leave to the hospitals to deal with.

♣ *Foreign Nurses*

To continue the example of nurses, the situation with foreign trained nurses is similar to that of the British trained nurses, except that it is the hospitals who attest to the NMC that they have verified that the foreign nurse job applicant is properly qualified and competent for registration. The motivation of the hospitals is based on government targets for safe staffing levels, and so **quantity** of staff is given precedence over **quality**. In the NHS, managers do not keep their jobs if they fail to meet targets, including those for staff levels, so they make up the numbers with anyone they can find.

As part of the interview and screening process for foreign nurses, the hospital or other NHS employer is expected to ensure that the applicant has the ability to communicate, in English, in the worst case scenario of a safety critical incident, such as with a trauma or cardiac arrest case. The employers meet this obligation to ensure language ability by accepting, from the applicant, a certificate of English language proficiency. Even with the certificates of proven language ability, many of these English proficient nurses (and doctors, etc) can only communicate by picking from a small number of commonly used key words and expressions – they speak a sort of tourist style pidgin English, but cannot ask or answer questions, and are unable to comprehend written information, such as patient histories.

Strikingly, if these people (with some rare exceptions) are present when an emergency occurs, they find reasons to absent themselves from the emergency. One example of this behaviour occurred at one London teaching hospital, when a surgical patient suffered a cardiac arrest, in the presence of a senior (band seven) anaesthetic nurse who, incidentally, achieved her well paid team leader status because of her "relationship" with a senior consultant surgeon. As soon as it became apparent that the patient had gone into cardiac arrest, this senior nurse quickly left the department, using the excuse that she had to retrieve a portable ECG machine from the Intensive Care Unit. When she returned, she stood to the side, gripping the ECG machine, as if associating herself with this piece of equipment would make it appear that she was on standby to perform an important and technical task. She made no attempt to become involved in the partaking or supervising of any aspect of the cardiac arrest protocol, such as is required of a band seven nurse, and she made no communication with any of the team members who were giving chest compressions, because she did not understand what was going on, or what was being said by the team members.

This incident shows how the nurse was not properly competent to undertake the duties required by the NMC and, to compound the issue, she did not have the English skills allowing her to understand the instructions and requests for help that emanated from the people involved in the cardiac arrest event. Her ability to act in the interests of the above vulnerable patient were virtually non existent.

The above account is not unique, and I have worked alongside NHS staff who have worked in the UK for over twenty years, who still cannot express their thoughts in English, in spoken or written form, or understand anything but the most basic things that others communicate to them ("tea break now", "where notes?" etc).

Naturally, these less than competent people gain no insight into those care and safety related things that are applicable to any particular patient's condition – they can only function in a manner that can be described as routine and predictable, and are unable to meet the professional and moral needs of behaving in either proactively or reactively safe ways.

* * *

Registration bodies like to claim that removing dangerous nurses and allied professionals from their registers is how they satisfy their mission to protect the public from harm, but it is they who allow these people to work as nurses (etc) in the first place, by enrolling them onto their registers - in return for annual registration subscription fees - but without taking even the most basic steps to ensure valid registration qualification and competency.

The rogue workers, such as the above, cannot be blamed for putting patients at risk. Their behaviour, though contrary to what is right and proper, is only a reflection of the type of people that they are which, in simple terms, is "unsuitable for delivering healthcare services". There should be a mechanism that prevents these rogue elements from being in positions where they have responsibilities for patient safety and welfare. That mechanism, clearly, should be the screening process that registration bodies fail to deliver.

Closing the stable door, after the horse has bolted, is the model that the registration bodies have adopted, but that does not meet the needs of a safe system of registration, neither does it comply with the *Precautionary Principle* imperative to assume that hazards will be realised, unless preventative measures are taken to mitigate against those hazards and, by doing so, reduce risk to patients.

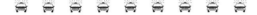

10: COVER-UPS & EMPLOYEES

The immediate aim of the cover-up culture is to suppress any information that could reflect badly on the part of the NHS, such as a particular hospital, that is responsible for a covering up an untoward event. By protecting the image of the hospital (for example), the status and reputation (and lucrative salary and benefits package) of the Chief Executive is also protected. Chief Executives, quite clearly, are incentivised to act against the openness and duty of candour that politicians like to claim are attributes of the NHS.

By minimising NHS "bad news", the sitting government gains a reputation for doing a good job of managing the NHS, and that ticks one of the major boxes for developing voter appeal. There are, however, implications for both staff and patients.

Patient Implications of the Cover-up Culture

The regular government inquiries into poor healthcare delivery, unsafe practices, high rates of unnecessary deaths, sepsis, and other examples of patients coming to harm, as a consequence of their treatment by the NHS, serve as a reflection of which parts of the NHS are failing their duty to the public. Unfortunately, it is only when information about negative NHS related events enter the public domain, via the press, that the government involve themselves in these events – it would be a vote loser if they did not appear to be concerned about whatever scandal is under scrutiny, so they have to make the right noises about how they are going to address whatever is of public concern. Before a particular issue becomes newsworthy, hospitals and NHS officials activate cover-up practices, and prolong them for as long as they are able. In the meantime, the public are unaware of the situation that poses a threat to their wellbeing, and they continue to be exposed to the poor treatment that ends up harming them. The clinical staff, who are aware of whatever dangers patient are subject to, can either speak out and report the dangers, and suffer insidious and escalating bullying and career damage, as a consequence, or they can cooperate with the cover-up practices that they know they are expected to comply with.

🚩 Employee Cooperation

Those issues that the NHS want to keep from the public cannot be concealed from NHS staff so, for the cover-up culture to work, the NHS needs the cooperation of the employees who know the truth about whatever is being concealed. By being part of any cover-up, the employees concerned have to compromise their registration duty to act in the best interests of patients; they contravene their duty under the Health and Safety at Work Act to minimise risk; they completely disregard the Health and Safety Executive requirement to comply with the Precautionary Principle, and they behave in opposition to both the NHS duty of candour, and the spirit of openness.

For the less able healthcare professionals, particularly the ones who have either cheated their way through their nursing (or Operating Department Practitioner etc) courses, are drug users (1 in 4), or possess fake qualifications, cooperating with management cover-ups is a sure route to job security and promotion. It is for this reason that the cover-up culture is so virulent, the rewards for the fakes, frauds, and drug users are generous and profligate.

Staff Implications of the Cover-up Culture

For those employees, from the most junior nurse, to the most senior Consultant, who fail to fall in line with the cover-up culture, and who, therefore, pose a threat to their employer's (Chief Executive) public status and job security, their reward is prolonged, persistent, and comprehensive personal and professional attacks. They will also be pushed into feeling isolated, and they will not be supported by professional bodies, or their colleagues. They have to fight the good fight on their own, and without the weapons to do so.

There is no such thing as an NHS management cadre who act on the concerns of a whistleblower, and nobody at director level will ever take steps to rectify whatever systemic faults need fixing, unless failing to do so puts their own position in peril. The concept of "patients first", which hospital public relations teams like to associate with the philosophies of their paymasters, is pure propaganda. The priority, everywhere in the NHS, is: ① Protect your job ② Protect your boss ③ Protect the Chief Executive ④ Protect the government.

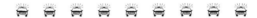

11: RECRUITMENT

At the most junior level (band five), a nurse or anaesthetic technician will perform their duties according to instructions and standard procedures, but will not be responsible for making anything other than trivial decisions concerning patient treatment. As the individual's career progresses, their knowledge and experience should be rewarded with promotion to higher bands and, with each promotion, their patient related decision making and responsibilities are increased. It is quite right that this should be the case, because junior staff do not have the authority or the requisite understanding of a patient's condition to determine courses of care, it would not be a safe way of working, so decisions should be left to more senior staff. Clearly, safe patient care is proportional to a healthcare practitioner's seniority. It follows from this correlation between seniority and safety, that recruitment and promotion should be determined in a way which coincides with the NHS Constitution directive - to ensure that staff are valued, and treated in a meritorious way, so that there is fair treatment and equal opportunity in recruitment and career development.

In reality, NHS recruitment and career development opportunities are based on favouritism, discrimination and, most significantly, the willingness of the individual to help enforce the cover-up culture.

Official NHS and hospital statements and policies, regarding equality and fairness, are really just frothy propaganda, designed to give the impression that the institution is being managed in the manner that the public expect.

Hear No Evil, See No Evil

When an NHS manager makes a written report, to their manager or director, of an important public interest or safety issue, that superior manager must deal with the problem, otherwise, if a related incident occurs, they will be held accountable for failing to take proper mitigating action, and they could lose their job. To protect against this scenario, the NHS has an unwritten law which requires that any "negative" information be kept from the relevant manager. In this way, should a problem occur, the manager can claim innocence, because they were not informed of the issue and, consequently, culpability passes down the food chain to whomever is the easiest to blame. NHS managers want to *see no evil and hear no evil* – as per the institutionalised concealment and cover-up culture of the NHS. If anyone in the management hierarchy does not comply with this unwritten law, they are unlikely to remain in post for long, and their chances for further promotion will be non-existent. So, they have to play ball, fit in with NHS politics, respect the **cover-up and protect your boss** culture, and "hear no evil, see no evil" at all times.

Departmental Managers

To maintain the above mentioned NHS "hear no evil, see no evil" mode of operating, a manager (with few exceptions) will employ and promote those who understand that their primary duty is to protect that manager. Similarly, the manager will appoint underlings, such as junior managers (band eight) and team leaders (band seven), whose loyalty to them is assured, will always act in their best interests, and above that which might be expected by professional registration requirements.

Members of the public may find it difficult to understand how a nurse manager - typically a matron - can depend on the corrupt loyalty of his or her subordinates. The answer to that is simple; many clinical (nurse etc.) promotions to band six and above are fraudulent, because those who are promoted are not competent or qualified for their new appointments. The proof of that fact lies in the knowledge and abilities of those promoted, including whether or not they are able to satisfy the competency requirements of their respective registration bodies (NMC, HCPC), particularly with respect to a knowledge of those areas of science and statistical analysis which form the core of healthcare practise. An even easier way to demonstrate lack of competency, particularly of a band seven (team leader) or band eight (manager or matron), is to determine whether or not they are able to satisfy the vitally important and mandatory registration requirement to be able to accurately and reliably solve relevant drug calculation problems – both basic and advanced types. It is quite usual for band five and band six staff to not have the ability to properly satisfy this drug calculation requirement, because it is a skill which is rarely called upon. For band seven/eight staff, the education, ability, and intelligence standards are, officially, at a much higher level. Staff at these bands are supposed to be educated to Master's degree level, and they are expected to be role models to more junior staff. In the NHS, the fraction of band seven and band eight nurses and anaesthetic technicians, who possess the appropriate science and numerical competencies, is probably less than one in a thousand, and that number is most likely limited to a small number of specialist areas, such as intensive care, emergency or advanced practitioner roles.

By being promoted to the senior and high paid level of band seven or eight, the undeserving and unqualified person's loyalty to their manager is assured, because they know that they can be justifiably demoted at the manager's whim, and they will have no recourse of redress to their demotion. Such loyalty to the manager supercedes commitment to ensuring the workplace is characterised by equal and fair treatment of staff, and ensures that only fellow supporters of the cover-up culture will experience career progress.

Recruitment Dirty Tricks

The NHS does not have viable controls or checks to ensure equal opportunities for recruitment, promotion, or other types of career development for employees, because these issues, ultimately, are at the whim of local managers and team leaders. The purpose of this short section is to demonstrate this fact, by listing a selection of unfair recruitment and promotion practices; it is not an exclusive list, just a sample of what happens.

♠ Party Girls
One corrupt recruitment practice is that of favouritism, where jobs

are given to those who can enhance the social lives of the person(s) responsible for their recruitment. In the private sector, this is unlikely to be of public concern, unless it presents a safety issue. In the NHS, however, the public expect people to be recruited and promoted according to their ability, potential, and meritorious service. Optimum healthcare, after all, is determined by the people who deliver the healthcare services, and optimum healthcare means optimum staff.

An obvious example of recruitment favouritism occurs at hospital T, where one particular anaesthetics team leader, Albert Steptoe (60 years old), would like, if he could get away with it, to only recruit young, blonde females, especially if they are newly qualified, or have the most basic ability or experience. The reason why he wants these young and naive girls in his team is obvious, and he boasts to his drinking pals that he has the "pick" of these girls, and has to take viagra to keep up with "demand".

The reason why he prefers to employ the least experienced and least capable girls (he refers to them as "his girls") is because they will always need support and rescuing from patient safety related situations which might otherwise cause them to lose their jobs and, possibly, their registrations. Whenever any of "his girls" needs help, they phone him (Albert), even if he is at home, and he comes to the rescue. His aim is to be their hero, so that they will more easily, and more gratefully, be absorbed into his social life, especially with regard to his Friday "team building" nights out, and Saturday night exotic parties. To the general public, this issue may seem almost innocuous, because it is just a case of a dirty old fopdoodle who is taking advantage of his position of authority to gain "favour" with some of the young females in his team. A little more analysis will shed a different light on the matter.

If Albert only employed the most gifted or experienced "young blondes", he would have nobody to rescue from work problems, and his social life would not benefit, because nobody would need his support, and there would be nothing for them to be grateful to him about. It follows that, because his policy is to recruit the least capable staff, he actively causes an increased risk to patients, and that is a contravention of his duty, under the Health and Safety at Work Act, to reduce risk to as low as reasonably practicable.

Another hospital T person who likes to employ "party girls", but for a different reason, is one of the department's managers (band 8 nurse) - Jill Pope. Jill knows that some of these young girls will be very "friendly" with some of the senior male doctors who they work with. Jill also knows that her position would be weakened if enough of these young blondes made negative comments about her, to those doctors. So, she uses the friendliness between the party girls and the doctors to her advantage, by developing the careers of these girls, putting them on the fast track to promotion, and allocating funds to put them on career enhancing courses. The manager (Jill Pope) also ensures that these favoured girls have their leave and shift requests approved, in preference to other staff, including those with child support needs. Jill knows that these party girls are then much more likely to say good things about her, to the doctors they are friendly with, and that will improve her professional standing. Essentially, she is using her position to allocate tax payer money to protect her job, rather than direct that money in a way that best serves patient care.

♣ Over Qualified

As in the rest of society, one often given reason to not recruit someone for a job in the NHS, is when the applicant is deemed to be "over-qualified". How anyone can be too qualified to do a healthcare job is nonsensical, and does not describe the true situation, which is that the manager or team leader, who asserts that the job applicant is overly qualified, is really saying that the applicant is better qualified than they are, and may become a competitive threat to their own position. This is the reverse meritocracy of the NHS in action. The situation can be perfectly exemplified by the behaviour of the senior anaesthetic technician (ODP) at Pilgrim Hospital, Boston, who left school at sixteen, with no qualifications, and who has an extreme prejudice to anyone who is more intelligent and educated than he is – which means most of society. His aversion to qualifications is realised by his recruitment policy, where he tries to disguise his prejudice by advising the better educated anaesthetic technician job and training applicants that they are over qualified, and should consider taking up medical (doctor) training instead. Proof of this matter can be found in the recruitment and promotion history of this anaesthetic technician's department, where he always recruits the least educated people.

♣ False Equality

When an employer, such as the previously mentioned Albert Steptoe (anaesthetics team leader) or Jill Pope (Department manager), preferentially employ people according to favouritism or discrimination, it will be very obvious what they are doing, but nobody dare raise the issue, lest they suffer career detriment. To guard against the possibility of being recognised as being guilty of such prejudice, a commonly used tactic, that occurs throughout the NHS, is for the manager to project the appearance of objectivity, by recruiting staff who they do not really want to employ and, by so doing, create the fiction of equality. This is the method used when recruiting the above mentioned "party girls". To illustrate:

If six people are recruited, and four are of the type - young, blonde, and not so bright "party" girls - favoured by the team leader (Albert Steptoe) or manager (Jill Pope), the remaining two "undesirables" will be recruited to help give the impression that the rules of equality and diversity have been followed. These people will be either male, Asian, black, older females, or highly educated with genuine qualifications, as opposed to the faux healthcare qualifications (M.Sc. etc) available in the UK. and they will suffer unfair treatment, and have no support in their roles. They will be made to feel uncomfortable and unwelcome, and when requesting any type of guidance or leadership for the jobs, they will be told, by Albert Steptoe: "Wot jexpect me ta do abaaht it? Sort it aaht yself!".

Albert will attempt to set these people up to fail, and to face criticism by colleagues, by putting them in stressful and demanding positions, where they need official support, which is not forthcoming, all with the intention of making them appear unsuitable for the promotion which he wants to reserve for "his girls", and making them unhappy enough to minimise their tenure at the hospital. Albert's aims, strategy, and tactics are blatant and persistent, and known by everyone in hospital T's Operating Theatre Department.

Another dirty trick, from Albert, is to help reduce the possibility that some of his party girls would be overworked, or might finish their day shifts late, particularly on Fridays, which is when his team enjoy their "team building" social nights with him. To achieve this, Albert regularly employs extra agency staff to do the work of one or more of the young blondes, and then assigns the "spare" girls to double-up with other young blondes. Essentially, Albert uses taxpayer's money to employ someone from an agency to do the work of one girl, so that she and another girl can share the workload which one person is supposed to have. This gives each girl a very easy and non-tiring day, and ensures they are fresh for their night out. This practice meets the definition of corruption, which other staff are aware of, but dare not report, lest they be set up to be disciplined.

To disguise the dearth of intelligence and ability in his team, Albert tried to compensate by spreading the rumour that other people were referring to his team as the "super team", and he tried to give the impression that the "super team" was exclusive to the best anaesthetic technicians (ODPs and nurses), none of whom had ever made mistakes - because Albert would always cover up for them.

Albert was not blessed with a normal ration of brain cells (cruel but true), and his remaining cells have been diminished by his lifestyle "habits" so his acumen and foresight were insufficient for his "super team" ruse, so it was inevitable that it was doomed to failure, and that happened when some of the scrub nurses starting referring to his "super team" as the "slapper team".

⚜ Interviews

In the NHS, the process of selecting job applicants is given the veneer of validity by conforming to the standard practice of aptitude testing in interview processes. In theory, only those who satisfactorily answer the given technical and procedural questions will be considered as having passed the interview. In practice, the decision who to employ is usually made beforehand, and the interview process is just a sham.

One way to justify an offer of employment to a preferred candidate is to ensure that person is given the interview questions and answers beforehand, so they do better than the other candidates. There is nothing revelational about this type of cheating, it is not exclusive to the NHS but, in the healthcare setting, failing to select staff according to ability, means that, once again, it is not the best staff who are employed, and the legal obligation (Health and Safety at Work Act) to reduce risk is contravened, because employing weak recruits gives senior staff, such as Albert, the opportunity to gain favour with them, because he constantly protects them from making mistakes and covering up for them.

♣ Nepotism

Nepotism is another issue which has a universal reach, and almost certainly occurs in all government institutions as much as it occurs in private industry. A graphic example of nepotism, in the NHS, is when a senior person, typically a nurse or doctor, arranges for a family member, such as a son or daughter, to find employment at their own place of work, usually as a healthcare assistant. Even more nepotistic, and fraudulent, is when the senior staff member uses their influence or authority to arrange for their child to be accepted onto the "secondment" scheme, which is where an unskilled member of staff is approved, after a qualifying one or two year period of employment, to be accepted onto a taxpayer funded training course to become a nurse, paramedic, or anaesthetic technician (Operating Department

Practitioner). Whilst on their course, the seconded student remains employed by the NHS, and continues to draw full pay and pension contributions.

The following table gives examples of secondment instances:

Hospital	Senior Staff	Relationship
Grantham	Theatre Department Manager (matron)	Son
Hammersmith	Doctor Kirby	Son
Lincoln	Senior Nurse	Daughter
St George's, Tooting	Jacqui Bishop, Anaesthetics Manager (matron)	Boyfriend (porter)

The total cost of a secondment training place is approximately £120,000 - £140,000 for the three years of studentship. Other students, of course, have to borrow large sums of money to fund their training. For most parents of grown up children, the problem of having to borrow money to fund their university place, and living expenses, is a source of great stress and anxiety, for them and their child. Not so for some senior hospital staff and their children.

Secondment is, quite clearly, a very generous scheme, which is available to very few people, and is another of the NHS's dirty secrets, and for good reason, because it is a corrupt use of power by NHS employees, and a fraudulent use of public funds.

♟ Employed To Fail

Another trick that managers use to justify appointing a loyal vassal to a senior position, without making it obvious that there is any favouritism in doing so, is to appoint someone else to that post, who the manager knows is doomed to fail, either because they are unsuitable for the job, or because they will be set up to fail. After a trial period of employment has shown that the appointee is unsuitable, the manager can replace that person with their preferred ally. In this manner, the appearance is given that the manager did not show any initial favouritism to their friend or vassal, and only brought them in when the first person proved incapable of filling that particular role.

♟ Interview Cheating

Job interviews are meant to filter out the poorest applicants, and to determine the best candidates for the job. In the NHS, interviews are often sham affairs, where the function of the interview is to give the impression that candidates are selected by an objective and competitive process. A common trick, as previously mentioned, to ensure that the favoured applicants are successful in their interviews, is to provide those applicants with the questions and answers in advance of their interviews. To provide extra assurance that those preferred applicants succeed at their interviews, the interviewers can introduce questions which most applicants would find difficult to answer, but which the favoured applicants are pre-warned about. Example questions include issues concerning the Lord Francis Report, government policies, clinical governance, and any other subjects not directly concerned with the job which the applicants are being interviewed for. Once the interview process is complete, the manager can justify their choice of applicants by using the results of the interviews and, by doing so, also help give the impression that the selection process has been based on merit.

♠ Preferential Recruitment from Poor Countries

NHS hospitals are zealous in their recruitment of nursing staff from poor countries, and managers will publicly sing the praises of those people, with such claims as "they are excellent nurses" and "the NHS would collapse without them". Nobody ever sings the praises of British nurses or allied professionals – there is no political or professional advantage in doing so, especially as saying anything positive about the British will be translated as being discriminatory against everyone else. The British are the only people who discriminate against themselves, and that is one reason why we are seen as a weak and feeble race – we hate ourselves, but embrace the rest of the world.

But why are NHS managers reluctant to recruit people from the United Kingdom, or from other developed countries? Also, why do hospitals pay (not lend) the air fares and first month's accommodation costs for staff from poorer countries, but won't pay the train fares or similar accommodation costs from staff moving from another part of the U.K., to live near the hospital? Why the unequal treatment? The answer to those questions is because of the NHS cover-up culture; third world staff are more willing to comply with the imposed practice of not raising issues because, if they do speak out about an issue of poor patient care, for example, they will become vulnerable to the retribution that would open up the possibility of them losing their right to stay in the U.K., so they concentrate on "fitting in", and tend not to speak out about anything that might produce negative press for the NHS, or the government.

At some hospitals, the preferential treatment for staff from the third world also extends to allocating hospital accommodation. This is a practice that serves to indirectly make it difficult for British nursing staff to be job mobile - especially if they want to work in a London hospital, where rental accommodation is unreasonably expensive and, frequently, unpleasant and dangerous. Managers, of course, will claim that they have to recruit from overseas, because they cannot find British staff to work in their hospitals.

At one large London hospital, British recruits are placed on long waiting lists for key worker accommodation, yet foreign non key workers, such as cleaners and drivers, who are not directly employed by the NHS, are allocated key worker rooms as soon as they become available. Another practice is to allocate the best accommodation, which are non-shared studios, to non-British staff only. If anyone complains about this or any other type of anti-British discrimination, they will be targeted with the enforcement component of the *NHS cover-up triad* – **bullying**.

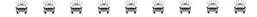

◨ 12: PROMOTION

As with the issue of recruitment, promotion in the NHS is not dependent on who is the best person for the job, but who best protects the manager's interests and job security. To ensure that promotion is restricted to those favoured by the manager, underhand and non-meritorious tricks are used, including:

◨ Disciplining Staff

An effective technique of ensuring that someone, who the manager does not like, is to make them seem unsuitable for promotion, by arranging for them to suffer disciplinary action, typically for the accusation of being aggressive. This is a common practice.

◨ Personal Relationships

As previously mentioned, a method to ensure promotion for an unworthy applicant, is for them to establish a "hanky-panky" type relationship with a senior member of staff - doctor, team leader, or manager. These relationships are very common, and are never successfully hidden from other staff, especially those overlooked for the promotion gained by the hanky-panky "practitioner".

⚙ Night Shifts

It has long been known that patient safety is lower at weekends and during night shifts, and one of the reasons for that is staff abandoning their posts to take part in amorous liaisons. Predictably, the culprits will be doctors meeting nurses.

When a nurse leaves his/her place of work, such as a surgical ward, to meet their "partner" in an office or store room, they are putting their patients at risk, because they are not observing them, or regularly recording their physiological values, and they cannot initiate emergency procedures **immediately** after a patient suffers, for example, a seizure or cardiac arrest, because they are absent. To satisfy the requirements of safety, it should always be the worst case scenario that clinical staff have to be prepared for, and that is only possible when staff are where they are supposed to be.

For the junior "partner" in the above described liaisons, such as a nurse, the benefit is enhanced job security and career progression (helped by the senior); for the senior "partner", typically a doctor, the benefit is considered one of the perks of the job.

⚙ Middle-aged Manager and Young Novice

A blatant example of undeserved promotion for a relationship occurred, predictably, at hospital T, described thus:

A newly qualified anaesthetic technician (early 20's) was recruited to work in the operating theatres department, some six months after failing his course, due to incompetence, and which he had to redo, until he was deemed to have passed his assessment criteria. During that pre-employment six months period, he had to undergo remedial training to get him through the acceptance criteria for the course, and the qualification for which he did not deserve.

Soon after starting work at Hospital T, he showed that he had a very minimalist and uncaring attitude to his duties, and he quickly gained a habit for failing to perform the basic stocking up, equipment checking, and "setting up" tasks that his role entailed, and he tended to take the short cut of taking stock and equipment from his colleagues. He was quickly marked down, by his peers, as being dangerous and untrustworthy. However, to his band eight manager (late 40's female matron), he was both physically and personally appealing; he had low morals, low intelligence, was brash, and exhumed a confident manner. He was the type of "bad boy" that she had a penchant for. Their relationship was established within the first few weeks of his employment.

During his first two years in the department, there were several occasions when this anaesthetic practitioner arrived at work not fully in control of his faculties (drugs). Arriving at work in such a condition should have resulted in disciplinary action, and being reported to his registration body, leading to suspension or loss of his registration. Not him – he was just sent home, for being "sick".

* * *

Immediately after completing the minimum two years of post qualifying service, this "favourite" of the manager was automatically promoted to band six, ahead of twenty or more other employees, some of whom had fifteen to thirty years more experience, and significantly more knowledge and ability than he. Nobody complained, of course, because that would have meant being put on the pathway to career destruction.

Six weeks after his promotion, his manager created a band seven position, for which he was the only applicant, so he would get the job.

For readers who are not aware of NHS bands, newly qualified nurses and allied professionals start at band five, senior staff (nursing "sister" or senior paramedic, etc) are at band six, team leaders are band seven, and bands eight and nine are classed as management. The education level for a band seven is that of Master's degree, or above, but this technicality was overlooked for this favourite of the manager; he left school with, as other staff liked to remark, only a GCSE in Woodwork (you get the drift).

Note: *Band seven is a significant jump from band six, and is a very desirable "rank" to have because, with few exceptions, they do not work night shifts, weekends, or on-call. A clinical band seven is supposed to have superior intellectual ability, leadership skills, and wealth of knowledge and experience, particularly with respect to dealing with clinical emergencies.*

For this "bad boy", moving from band five to band seven meant a giant leap in rank, for which he was both unsuited and unqualified, to the dizzying heights of the assumed persona of one with both a superior intellect, and superior ability. His case is not unique.

Promotion Dirty Tricks

♨ Tactical Promotion

When a manager wants justification for promoting a favoured staff member, there are two well used tactics for ensuring that the "right" person gets the promotion. One way is to ensure that training budget funds are used to put the favoured person on appropriate job enhancing training courses whilst, simultaneously, using the excuse of lack of funds to prevent other staff from attending those same training courses. When the job is advertised, the selection criteria will stipulate experience and qualifications that match those of the manager's favoured employee, making them the only candidate suitably qualified for the promotion.

Another trick, which is often effectively hidden from scrutiny, is where rules and policy statements prevent some people from being promoted, but are over-ridden, or worked around, to allow others to bypass those rules and policies. A common example is that of an employee who switches from permanent to so called "bank" employment, which means that the worker becomes a temporary employee, and has the ability to match their working hours to their personal circumstances. Many bank employees work as many shifts as permanent staff, and do so for many years but, because the rule is that a bank employee cannot be promoted, they have no career progression. That is, unless they have a "special" relationship with their team leader or manager, in which case, justification is created to bend the rules so that the bank worker is given promotion.

🔊 Tactical Promotion

Hospitals decree how many people there can be, in each department, and at particular bands (ranks). When a manager wants to prevent promotion for a particular employee, they can do so by promoting someone less deserving and, thereby, ensure that the more senior posts are all occupied. The more deserving employee cannot then claim discrimination is stopping them from being promoted, because it is the hospital, not the manager, who decides how many people there can be at particular bands.

🔊 Job References

References are a throwback to the master/servant days, when a domestic worker sought employment with an upper class family who did not want to employ anyone who could not be trusted to keep confidential family information. For assurance, they would trust a written reference from the applicant's previous employer, another upper class family. Giving a false reference would be an ungentlemanly thing to do, so references were taken as being reliable.

Providing job references has developed into de rigueur practice in the modern age; employers ask for them because that is the fashion. The reference serves as a tool that the potential employer uses as an extension of their power over the job applicant – it is a form of non-aggressive but intrusive interrogation, which has no positive or practical effect. Indeed, the authenticity of a reference's contents are guided by personal feelings of the referee; if they are on friendly terms with the job applicant, they will produce a good reference; if the referee is keen to be rid of the job applicant, either for personal or professional reasons, they will provide an even better reference, in the hope that the reference will win the unwanted employee the new job. In the NHS, references are a universally adopted method of controlling staff, who might otherwise let their managers know how they feel about them, and the hospital. How, for example, would an employee gain a fair and accurate reference from their manager, when the reason they are seeking new employment is because they have blown the whistle about the manager's disregard of safety, drug use, or fraud? (References is one of the methods which the NHS uses to coerce staff into compliance with the cover-up culture.)

♨ Feigned Equality for Promotion

Another technique that a manager can use to prevent a non-favoured employee from being promoted, whilst giving the impression that they are acting in the employee's best interests, is to encourage that employee to apply for promotion, after they have already lined up another person for the promotion.

When the employee is unsuccessful at their interview, the manager may feign disappointment, and try to make the employee think that they are just as disappointed as the employee is. In reality, the dual purpose of encouraging the employee to apply for a job that they would never get, is to convey the impression that the interview process is based on fairness and equality, and to cause embarrassment to the employee, so that they will be discouraged from making further applications, because the possibility of a second failure would be too embarassing and unbearable to contemplate.

⚓ 13: STAFF DISCRIMINATION

Discrimination, in its various forms, is something which occurs in all parts of the world, including the United Kingdom where, compared with most other countries, it is mostly of a tame nature. Any serious cases of discrimination, in the U.K., especially where violence occurs, are very rare, so much so that they attract national publicity. In modern Britain, discrimination is considered an unproductive and unacceptable characteristic of a peaceful society, and some types of discrimination are deemed a criminal offence, as detailed by the Equality Act (2010).

Curiously, the introduction of the Equality Act has had no effect on age discrimination and, more curiously, since the 1970's, anti-British and anti-English discrimination, which is growing with increasing invidiousness. We now have the situation, in many industries, especially the NHS, where being English, in England is, in fact, a disability. This is especially so for working class English males – the middle and upper classes are mostly immune from this problem, in fact, they are often the cause of it. Working class English males, it seems, only have value when, as they say, "there is a war on". (The same can be said of the rest of the United Kingdom)

General Discrimination

In the NHS, discrimination is more pronounced than it is in general society, with anti-British (especially anti-English) and anti-male discrimination being the most prevalent of the demographics. Anti-female discrimination also occurs, of course, especially against those females who are more likely to advocate for patient safety, and raise issues where appropriate – they threaten the cover-up culture, so they are seen as threats to managers.

The easiest way to illustrate the relevance of the varied characteristics is with the following table illustrating, in each row, which of two hypothetical candidates, who are in competition for employment or promotion, and who are similar in every way, except for one discriminatory factor, is successfully employed or promoted. For example, the second line shows that when a British and non British candidate compete for a position, the non British candidate is more likely to be successful.

♨ General Discrimination Factors

Favoured	*Discriminated*
Sycophantic. Loyal to cover-up culture.	Non-obsequious. Loyal to patient care.
Non British	British
Female	Male

Favoured	*Discriminated*
Younger	Older
Uneducated	Educated
Dim	Intelligent
Alcoholic	Sober
Drug user	Anti-drugs

The last two lines (Alcoholic, Drug user) may not occur as commonly as the other discriminants, but they have been included, because they are relevant at hospital T, for example, where they are used as controlling factors of the drug users, by managers, to ensure loyalty and compliance with the cover-up practices of the hospital.

As for the remaining factors, they will be applied in various combinations, and to varying degrees, in almost all NHS places of employment. If this were not the case, I would be foolish to make such an assertion, but the evidence, as I have previously stated, is there, if any objective body cares to look.

Specific Discrimination

In addition to the above NHS universal rules of discrimination, particularly against English males or older females, there are, quite predictably, other types of discrimination which are specific to particular NHS managers and establishments.

🕮 Discrimination Claims

For balance with the section following this, I have to mention that some employees with protected titles (religion, race, etc.), particularly in unskilled roles, will make false allegations of discrimination, as a defence against disciplinary action for not doing their jobs properly. This is a well known and well worn tactic which, because of its overuse, is losing its credibility, and is less effective than it once might have been, but it is still a tactic of choice or, perhaps, of last resort. Such false claims of discrimination are commonly seen as "get out of jail" cards, and are easy to make, because there are no repercussions for making them.

🕮 Genuine Discrimination

Noticeably, for black clinical staff in one particular hospital, apparent discrimination is as obvious as it is against the English but, unlike unskilled employees, clinical workers are much less likely to complain about being discriminated against, and not because they are unlikely to be believed. The main reason for the reluctance to speak up is because employees know that senior staff, and personnel department clerks, have no reservations in assembling disciplinary cases against them, with fake allegations of professional transgressions, such as aggression against colleagues. NHS employees may not understand the bullying methods that might be used against them, but they are aware that "dirty tricks" are NHS tools of the trade to close down any issue, such as a claim of discrimination or favouritism, which has the potential to generate adverse publicity, and might weaken the cover-up culture of the NHS. Those dirty tricks, incidentally, can also include action taken by the victim's registration body which, for nurses, is the Nursing and Midwifery Council (NMC), and for Allied Professions is the Health and Care Professions Council (HCPC). Disciplinary action, by a registration body, can result in suspension or complete cancellation of the victim's registration and, hence, remove their right to continue working in their profession. Loss of registration is a Sword of Damocles hanging over professionally registered staff, and NHS managers use this to their cruel advantage.

What drew my attention to how blatant discrimination can be, in the NHS, was a series of incidents at St George's Hospital (Tooting), which occurred within a few months of a new anaesthetic team manager (band eight nurse) settling into her post. As with her predecessor, the new manager had no knowledge or experience of anaesthetics nor, indeed, had she ever worked in an operating theatre. Her lack of knowledge about the work that her team members did meant that she did not involve herself in any relevant technical, clinical, leadership, training, or procedural issues. Instead, she concentrated on being oppressive and threatening, to intimidate her team into not raising issues which might be of interest to the public, or might prove embarrassing for the hospital. That was what she was recruited to do.

Black Nurse 1

Shortly after assuming her new post, the anaesthetics team manager she decided to set an example of ruthlessness, by disciplining a black nurse, who failed to complete a mandatory administrative task, prior to the start of her surgical list. The punishment the nurse was given was as harsh as it could be, and included demotion, reduction in seniority and pension rights, and significant embarassment for her. The nurse was, indeed, guilty of a failure in her duties, but there were mitigating circumstances for her failure, inasmuch as the surgeon sent for the first patient, before the nurse was ready for the list to start. It is also of note how differently some other staff are treated, when they make similar or worse mistakes. In this manager's particular team, there are a relatively high number of staff who the rest of the department describe as "young blonde females", not all of whom are actually blonde, and not all are so young - ages range between twenty-one and mid thirties - but they are referred to as young blondes because that is the penchant of the anaesthetic technician team leader who recruits them, and for several of the surgeons and anaesthetists who enjoy "working" with them.

Whenever one of the young blondes fails to complete some similar task which the black nurse was disciplined for, no action is taken against them, because there is never a case to answer. This is because the young blonde's immediate action, for making this or any other error, is to inform the team leader, who comes to the rescue by, for example, hiding or falsifying official documentation in order to remove evidence of the problem. This is his "knight in shining armour" mode, and some of his girls are very "grateful" for it.

Within a year or so of the above incident, two other black nurses suffered disciplinary action, both of which were for false allegations. These cases were designed to protect other nurses, who were guilty of misconduct, by scapegoating the two black nurses:

♣ Black Nurse 2

This incident was one which had serious implications for patient safety, because it involved a "young blonde" anaesthetic nurse, Alaina Onatopp, whose aberration of her moral and professional duties, during a night shift, caused a risk to a patient's safety, when she failed to carry out her responsibilities to set up an operating theatre for a cardiac emergency, and to organise an additional "on-call" anaesthetic nurse to deal with that emergency. Instead of complying with her professional obligations, the nurse (Alaina Onatopp) passed the problem onto another anaesthetic nurse, who was middle aged and black, and who was responsible for dealing with emergency cases in a different wing of the hospital. Her (the black nurse's) obligations were defined by the department's published protocols for night shift anaesthetic staff, which prohibited her from abandoning her post, lest she become unavailable for her assigned place of work, which was the emergency operating theatre.

As a consequence of Alaina Onatopp's (young blonde) attempts to pass on her duties to the black nurse, there was a delay in treating the patient, and the delay meant increased risk to that patient. The surgeons, quite reasonably, were most unhappy about the delays in tending to the emergency patient, caused by absence of anaesthetic technicians, and they wanted the matter properly investigated.

Any investigation, in the NHS, means someone will be blamed for whatever the issue is, and a junior employee is always blamed – managers never assume culpability. The chance of a clinical manager, taking the blame for anything that a junior staff member can be blamed for, is unheard of – it just doesn't happen. In this instance, the blame was all on the part of the first nurse, Alaina Onatopp (young blonde), but it was the black nurse who experienced disciplinary action, and who was found guilty of putting the patient's life at risk. What made this incident noteworthy, and which drew my attention, were four things:

Firstly, the young blonde nurse, Alaina Onatopp, was from the same country as the manager, and they were friends.

Secondly: Two black nurses were disciplined within the space of just a few months, yet none of the gang of young blonde nurses were ever disciplined, or suffered any sanction which would injure their career development.

Thirdly: The black nurse defended herself by providing verifiable proof of her account of events, and other proofs which showed that the young blonde nurse had fabricated information to make it appear that she was innocent of wrongdoing. In addition, the black nurse proved that she had acted properly, and in accordance with the department's official protocols for night shift responsibilities.

The disciplinary panel consisted of the personnel department's chief "prosecutor", the team manager, and the appointed case manager (band seven ODP), who was the anaesthetic team practice educator. None of the panel considered or even accepted submissions provided by the black nurse, which is a contravention of a rule of natural justice - to make decisions based on evidence.

Fourthly: After the black nurse was found guilty of unprofessional and dangerous behaviour, the Theatre Department Manager changed the anaesthetic team's night shift protocols, so that it best matched the guilty verdict against the black nurse. Lawyers, undoubtedly, would say that this retrospective changing of conditions is both outrageous and scandalous. Such is the parallel universe of the National Health Service!

> If members of the public would like to know why patient safety is degraded at weekends and during night shifts, one prominent factor could be that senior staff – team leaders (band seven) and managers (band eight) – do not work at these times, or any other anti-social times, so rebellious staff can run riot. Incidentally, during night shifts, surgical procedures are all of an emergency nature but, even so, senior staff are never present at such times.

♣ Black Nurse 3

One problem, which rarely involves nurses, is that of violence between colleagues. Most nurses are tuned to their professional duties, and to their responsibilities towards patients, and aggression between nurses would be most rare and unexpected.

At St George's hospital, one nurse, Ludmilla Wournos (white), was transferred from a ward to the operating theatre department, as a punishment for persistent aggressive behaviour towards other members of staff. One day, whilst tending to a patient who was recovering from a surgical procedure, Wournos decided that she deserved a break, so she instructed a fellow nurse (black), who also had a patient to tend to, that she must take over her duties, so that she could have a rest. The black nurse informed Wournos that she could not abandon or pass on the responsibility for her patient, unless she was formally relieved by a colleague. The response from Wournos was to slap the black nurse in the face; she (black nurse) immediately reported the incident to the hospital's security team, and then phoned her manager, and informed her that she (black nurse) intended to call the police. The anaesthetics team manager persuaded the black nurse not to call the police, and let her deal with the issue instead. When the manager arrived, she spoke with Wournos (slapper), in their own language (E European), and calmed the situation, or so it seemed.

The following day, the black nurse received a letter from the personnel department, informing her that she was to be the subject of disciplinary action for her aggressive behaviour towards the manager, and for making up the story that she had been slapped by nurse Wournos. The black nurse informed the personnel department that they had made a mistake, and she had witnesses to prove that she was the one who was the victim. However, when she spoke to the nurses (Filipina/os) who witnessed the incident, they all denied knowledge of what happened. This was not surprising, because the other nurses knew that their own futures were best served by complying with the "Hear no evil, see no evil" behaviour required by the hospital. Subsequently, the black nurse was found guilty of the charges brought against her. The slapping nurse, Wournos, did not face any sanction, either officially, or unofficially.

In summary, in this particular department, and over the course of approximately one year, three black nurses suffered disciplinary action and, collectively, it was three nurses from one particular country who caused these disciplinary actions to occur. This does not necessarily mean that these cases were definitely a result of racist or any other kind of discrimination but, to paraphrase a British legal concept, a reasonable man might conclude that to be the case.

🖘 Hammersmith Hospital

Hammersmith Hospital is worth a specific mention, because its significant staff shortage problem, both permanent and agency, is so highly influenced by its discrimination and favouritism practices.

♣ Discrimination & Favouritism

In the Operating Theatre Department, none of the senior staff are male. The managers (band 8 nurses) are female, as are all of the team leaders and clinical practice educators (band 7). A male will only be appointed to a band 7 position if no female can be found to fill the role, and even then only if it is a temporary post. This anti-male discrimination is not unusual in the NHS, indeed, it is standard practice, and stems from the fact that a female manager will always find it easier to be domineering and threatening towards female staff, such is the character of the NHS version of leadership.

At the other end of the scale, the few token male clinical staff are all at the lowest pay band - band 5 - even though these people (anaesthetic technicians) are the most experienced staff in the department. Keeping these male members of staff at the lowest band can be likened to a football manager making the best players play in the reserve team – it is counter-productive. However, it is reflective of the degree to which the NHS respects the concepts of equality, quality, and meritorious service, which is virtually nil.

Another discriminatory factor that is most prominent in Hammersmith Operating Theatres, is that of its anti-British fervour. The anaesthetics team, for example, has a manager from an Eastern European country, and her anti-Britishness is impossible to disguise. Her recruitment policy matches the model for most NHS employers, which is is based on who best protects her position, and not on who is best for the job. To that end, her policy is to maximise employment of Eastern Europen females, and fill the remaining posts with "anyone but the British", which means other foreign females and, if reliably sycophantic ones can be found, Eastern Europen males.

⊟ 14: FAVOURITISM

Favouritism is an ubiquitous characteristic of the NHS, which governs promotion and other career development opportunities for staff of all disciplines and grades. Favouritism conflicts with the requirements of a safety culture, because it nullifies group values. By inference, those who practice favouritism are in breach of safety legislation (Health And Safety At Work Act), which is a criminal offence, punishable by six months in prison, and an unlimited fine, so it is a serious matter.

This short section presents samples of how favouritism is realised in the NHS, and illustrates how the concept of equality is advertised as being a valued NHS behaviour when, in reality, it is a propaganda topic, designed to reflect the institution as being law abiding, moral, and meeting with public expectations.

⊟ Losing Controlled Drugs

One of the roles of an anaesthetic technician, or an anaesthetic nurse, is to manage the safe storage, issuance, and recording of controlled drugs, such as Morphine, Cocaine, and Diamorphine (heroin). Sometimes, especially during extraordinarily stressful workloads, the technician or nurse can lose track of the drugs they administered, and the stored balance might not match the written record of drugs issued. In such instances, the details have to be reported, and an investigation must be undertaken, to discover the reason for the discrepancy. If the discrepancy is not resolved, management can class such a problem as a case of human error, or it can be considered a reportable offence, in which case there will be involvement of the pharmacy department and, in some cases, the police, and prosecution may ensue. Misplacing a controlled drug, therefore, can be a career destroying incident. However, if the person who misplaced the drug is a "friend" of the relevant team leader or manager, the incident can be white-washed by official trickery, and the whole matter can be buried. This is something that does happen, as described thus:

At hospital T, when a member of one particular anaesthetic team, led by the prolific scoundrel of an anaesthetic technician, Albert Steptoe, "loses" a controlled drug, the action taken is dependent on who "lost" the drug. If it is one of Albert' party girls, he rescues them from potential disciplinary action by making an entry into the controlled drugs register - a legal document - that the missing drug ampoule was, in fact, administered and opened, but returned unused, or the ampoule was dropped and broken.

The pharmacy audits of drug cupboard contents do not verify that drug administration entries are properly made, they only check that the balance in the register matches the count in the drug cupboard. When Albert protects his young blondes, by recording that the ampoules were broken or wasted, he contravenes the Misuse of Drugs Act (1971) but, as always, the NHS cover-up culture allows him to go unpunished – because he supports that culture.

⚜ Promotion

Promotion as a result of favouritism is one of the greatest causes of ill-feeling in the NHS, and it is something that occurs, most probably, in every department of every hospital; it is part of the fabric of NHS behaviour; it is as institutionalised as the NHS cover-up culture itself, and that is why it crops up in a number of chapters of this book, particularly in Chapter 12, *Promotion,* where the sections on *Relationships* and *Tailored Promotion* portray the reality of how much NHS career development is determined by favouritism and personal relationships.

⚜ Surgeon Blames Nurse

Lack of equality is endemic in the NHS, with one example being the practice of making scapegoats of junior staff, and protecting favoured and more senior staff, when something goes wrong. The following account describes how a senior member of staff, in this case, a surgeon, escaped scrutiny and sanction for causing an incident that placed a patient in danger, by using a nurse as a scapegoat for the surgeon's greed and recklessness.

The incident occurred in an operating theatre, where fifteen children where scheduled for general surgery. Those cases should have been scheduled over two days, but the surgeon wanted to complete them in one day, so that she could have the following day off, to moonlight in a private hospital.

Preparation for a surgical procedure requires a lot of retrieving, setting up, and checking of equipment and instruments. Between procedures, instruments have to be cleared away and sent for sterilisation, nurses have to decontaminate equipment and surfaces, including the floors (outsourced cleaners won't clean theatre floors), then the next case has to be prepared for. Additional work, which is ongoing, is filling out forms and documents. The "nurse in charge" ensures that tasks are properly performed. In this particular instance, the "nurse in charge" was in fear of the surgeon, who is renowned for her hostility towards nursing staff, and the damage she can do to the career of anyone who does not kowtow to her every whim (so much for the British sense of fair play and equality). The surgeon did not see herself as being part of a team who, collectively, delivered a service to patients but, instead, saw herself as solely delivering the service to patients, and considered the theatre team as being service providers to her - not the patient, which is in complete contradiction with NHS and registration body (NMC, HCPC) descriptions of service delivery . She, the surgeon, did not want to hear about team issues, such as equipment or staff shortages, and it was of no concern to her that, for example, there were only three out of the usual five theatre staff available, or that the hospital had stopped buying the surgeon's favourite instruments, and she had to use ones from an inferior supplier. No! For this surgeon, every problem was the fault of the "service providers" – the nurses, anaesthetists, and anaesthetic technicians (ODPs), and she made certain that everyone knew it was their fault. As far as the surgeon was concerned, everything had to happen exactly how and when she wanted, as if by magic, and there were no excuses. For the "nurse in charge", and the rest of the theatre team, concentrating on their jobs, whilst under the lash of this surgeon, was often sickeningly (literally) distracting and stressful.

To complete the fifteen surgical cases, the surgeon's communication with the theatre team was tinged with more than her usual level of bullying, disrespect, unreasonable demands, complaints, and threats. All the while, hinting that members of the team could be reported for being slow, or of lacking competency. By her behaviour, the surgeon increased the already inordinately high level of stress amongst the team, which is a well known factor in raising the probability of mistakes being made, and increasing the risk to the patients. This is, indeed, what happened.

Before commencement of the second case, one member of the team was sent to work in another theatre, because of her particular skills, and she was replaced by another nurse, who was told to scrub up for the current procedure (second case), quickly, because the surgeon was waiting for her to get ready. When the nurse arrived at the operating table, she asked if the sterile instrument tray had been properly checked, and if the counts of instruments and consumables was correct – she was told yes, the checks had already been done, and "Get on with it!". The surgeon, predictably, complained about the time lost due to the change of staff, and she wanted everyone to know that heads would roll, if she could not finish all of the cases on the list. The surgeon was not interested in safety procedures, or standard pre-surgical checks, she expected everything to be just so, and without having to request things – everyone had to be a mind reader.

Nobody, of course, dared speak out about the oppressive attitude of the surgeon, or of the bad atmosphere in the room; questioning the surgeon's running of the operating theatre would be like confronting a medieval queen, the result would have been the modern equivalent of "off with their head!".

Before the surgeon made the first incision into the child's skin, the replacement nurse noticed that some of the sterile instruments appeared contaminated. The tray, quite obviously, was from the previous case.

(*Using a contaminated surgical instrument on one patient, a so called* **never event**, *is almost certain to cause a potentially lethal infection in the second patient.*)

When the nurse drew the attention of the rest of the team to this issue, it became apparent that, in the confusion and panic of the change of staff, and the poor communication between the team, because of the surgeon's constant "cracking the whip", verbal abuse and complaints, nobody had packed up the instrument tray from the previous case, it was just put to the side, whilst everyone got on with other tasks. In the under-staffed, confused and oppressive atmosphere of the occasion, someone then assumed it was the tray for the second case. Events flowed from there.

Experienced scrub staff would say that this team was poorly managed, and not having a new sterile instrument tray was the responsibility of the nurse in charge, not the surgeon. That is easy to say, but safety experts would say that this was an avoidable safety issue, which occurred because the recipe (Swiss cheese model) for a failure of safety was consolidated by the one sided, accusatory, and aggressive demands from the surgeon, who was solely responsible for the poor atmosphere and poor communication that existed.

There was no investigation into this "never event"; instead, the surgeon complained about the replacement nurse who, shortly afterwards, was formally blamed and punished for failing to check the instrument tray. This automatic protection of the surgeon, and the redirection of blame and accusation of incompetence towards the nurse ("dead cat" strategy), illustrates how favouritism to one person has a corresponding negative affect on someone else. Favouritism, clearly, does not promote equality, safety, staff morale, or safe staffing levels. The nurse was disciplined and found guilty of safety violations, and she nurse handed in her notice a few weeks later.

♣ Moonlighting Surgeons

The above description of a surgeon "making" the time to work in a private hospital is not a unique case. For most surgeons, earning £150,000 p.a. from the NHS does not satisfy their lifestyle needs, so, moonlighting in private hospitals, with the prospect of raising their pay to approximately £250,000 is de rigeur practice. Surgeons might say that what they do in their own time is irrelevant to their employment by the NHS. In theory, this sounds quite reasonable. However, their NHS and private jobs are not discrete activities – they are closely linked. To illustrate, take the example of an NHS surgeon who works full time for an NHS hospital, and for a private hospital at weekends and on Friday and Monday evenings. (This surgeon's wife criticised me on Twitter, because I revealed how some surgeons will rush through their NHS cases, so that they have spare days available for private work - (moonlighting).

♣ Weekend Work

In this particular instance, the surgeon's main job (week days) is at an NHS hospital as a substantive employee – not a locum - and, unless he is otherwise engaged, he also works at a nearby private hospital, with appointment times advertised on his website as Saturdays, Sundays, and from 5.30 pm on Friday and Monday evenings.

To start an operation at the private hospital, at 5.30 pm, he will have to complete his list of, say, five NHS cases, by 3.30 pm, so that he can complete his paperwork for that day's cases, have a short meal break (required by Welfare at Work Regulations), travel to the private hospital, and meet the team for pre-surgery preparations and briefings. To ensure punctuality, he will plan his NHS list of cases so that they have reasonably predictable start times and durations, with the first case commencing at the standard time of 8 am.

Unfortunately, even though different patients may be similar in many ways, individuals are unique, and unexpected difficulties do occur with some of those individuals, and those differences invariably demand changes in techniques and/or equipment than what was expected and planned for. Those differences, naturally, can increase operating times, with the result that the finishing time for the case list will usually be extended. In such an instance, which is not so rare, the surgeon will have to make a choice between cancelling/postponing his last (fifth) case at the NHS hospital, so that he can be punctual for the cases at the private hospital, or finish all of the NHS cases, and cancel/postpone the cases at the private hospital. If the last NHS patient is cancelled and rescheduled, but the surgeon still reaches his target of cases numbers, the cancelled case is treated as just "one of those things", and there will be no repercussions to him. Alternatively, if he cancels one of the private hospital cases, that would result in both a cash flow hit, and reputational loss for the private hospital, with the result that the surgeon will be replaced.

At this point, I will leave the above description of how NHS and private care are inter-related, for the reader to ponder and calculate whether or not most surgeons will be more likely to sacrifice their lucrative private work, by giving priority to NHS patients.

✉ Favouritism & Discrimination

The following table gives examples of the types of favouritism and discrimination that characterise operating theatre departments in a selection of NHS hospitals (*scores 1-5, with 1 being the worst*).

Hospital	*1 = most favoured*	*1 = most discriminated*
Boston Pilgrim	1.Poorly educated 2.Locals	1.Graduates 2.Experienced
Charing Cross	1.Filipinos 2.Foreign females	1.British 2.Males 3.ODPs
Epsom	1.Females	1.Male 2.British
Grantham	1.Manager's family 2.Females	1.Educated 2.Males 3.ODPs
Guys Day Surgery	1.Asian females 2.Asian males 3.Other females	1.Hetero males 2.British 3.Black 4.ODPs
Guys Main	1.European females 2.Other females	1.British males 2.British females 3.Other males
Hammersmith	1.East European females 2.East European males 3.Other foreign females	1.British 2.Black/Asian 3.Males 4.ODPs
Kingston	1.Females	1.ODPs 2.Males 3.Black
Royal Free	1.Females 2.Foreign	1.Males 2.British 3.ODPs

Royal London	1.Foreign 2.Females	**1.British 2.Males**
Royal National Throat, Node, Ear **(Dr Patel)**	1.Females	**1.British**
St George's, Tooting	1.Young E European females 2.Older European females 3.Young non English UK females 4.Young English females 5. Older Non English UK females 6.Older English females 7.Asian females 8.Drug users 9.Fraudulently qualified	**1.Intelligent 2.Properly qualified 3.Males 4.English 5.Black**
UCL Main	1.Filipino females 2.Other foreign females 3.Filipino males	**1.British 2.Males 3.ODPs**
UCL Westmoreland St	1.Lesbians 2.Other females 3.European	**1.Males 2.Heterosexual 3.ODPs**
Whittington	1.Filipinos 2.Other Asians	**1.British 2.European 3.Black males**

🖾 Preference for Sychophants

In addition to the above personal characteristics of favouritism and discrimination, individual personality plays a more specific role, because it is the degree to which an employee poses a threat to the relevant departmental manager that supercedes all other considerations for how they are treated; if the manager considers a particular employee to be a strong enough character to speak out about issues of patient safety, and is not likely to be intimidated into keeping quiet about such matters, then that employee will suffer various threats to their career and work related social relationships.

Usually, the manager will ensure that the employee, who is considered a threat to the cover-up culture, is subject to indirect bullying tactics, including subtle and subliminal methods, which might be difficult to prove; for example: being socially excluded and ignored by colleagues who are subservient lackeys to the manager, being denied specific holiday or shift requests, being placed in unpopular work roles, including being made to work with people who may naturally discriminate against them, and any other method that will make life difficult and unpleasant for the victim.

Managers want employees who are sycophants, and employees who are most likely to be sycophantic are those who lack the ability to make career progress in a meritorious manner – their job security is dependent on their being sneaks and snitches, and acting as proxy bullies for their managers.

📋 Favouritism Ploy

As a measure of the widespread naivety amongst NHS staff, there is a commonly used trick that managers use to remove someone from their post, without that person realising what is being done to them, until the "removal" has been completed; described thus: When a manager wants to recruit or promote one on their friends, fellow countrymen etc, to a particular post, the person already in that post will be invited to apply for a temporary transfer, of a year or so, to a very appealing job that, on the surface, appears to be a career enhancing move, with special training, benefits, and such like.

Once the target person has accepted the temporary assignment, the manager's favoured person takes up that person's position which, again, is officially of the temporary type. However, once the target's temporary post has come to an end, the manager finds an excuse to prevent them from resuming their original position and, instead, offers them another position which, predictably, is an undesirable one, so they resign. (*Why victims do not recognise this trick is difficult to understand, because it is such a popular ploy.*)

15: DISCIPLINARY ACTION

O ne of the many unpleasant aspects of working in the NHS is the threat of disciplinary action. If an employee intentionally and maliciously does something which causes suffering or loss to individuals, disrupts processes, steals or causes damage to equipment or resources, then that person should, quite reasonably, suffer some sort of sanction, after they have been definitively proved guilty of the charges made against them.

Justice for NHS Employees

In reality, the problem is that many innocent employees, particularly those who speak out about patient safety, are disciplined, because they pose a professional or personal threat to their superiors, particularly their line managers. The reason why this is such a widespread problem, is because disciplinary action is a successful and easily implemented method to stifle and intimidate employees. Why disciplinary action, for false accusations, is so popular, is down to the fact that the NHS acts as a law unto itself, and the normal rules of natural justice and human rights are disregarded, and that gives NHS managers free rein to accuse and punish an employee of any offence they wish, however extreme, and the employee has no recourse to the normal protection that the law provides.

Disciplinary Action as a Deterrence

Unfair or ill found disciplinary action has, quite generally, the aim of frightening employees and deterring them from taking the route of "speaking out" about any issue which could be of patient safety or public interest, or which might otherwise prove embarrassing to the employer. This sort of intimidation is prolific in the NHS, and is one of the reasons why so many employees suffer long term stress and mental health problems, to the extent that they are not able to complete their planned career tenures.

Punishment

Once someone suffers disciplinary action, their personal standing with colleagues is permanently damaged, and their career prospects are quashed. Most significantly, if a manager wants to severely punish an employee, and set an example to other employees of what happens if they are not suitably submissive, disciplinary action can be followed by the killer blow of reporting the employee to their registration body, which is the General Medical Council for Doctors; Nursing and Midwifery Council for nurses; the Health and Care Professions Council for Paramedics, Biomedical Scientists, Radiographers, Anaesthetic Technicians (ODPs), and others.

Registration Bodies

Registration bodies will always tend to believe a case against the accused employee, and will only withhold their own sanctions, which include the suspension or loss of registration, if they cannot present a case which would stand up to scrutiny in civil court. A psychologist (Twitter @Penbat1) informed me that this **authority bias**, where belief is automatically assumed to come from the more powerful party, such as en employee's manager, is also a common occurrence with judges and the police, so the prejudice against an employee is systemic, deep rooted, and difficult to defeat.

If the situation were reversed, and the employee wanted to report the employer (hospital) to the employer's analogous overseeing body, which is the Care Quality Commission (CQC), they would not be entitled to trigger an investigation of the employer, or receive any type of support, and would not receive protection against retaliation from that employer. For the CQC to launch any proper investigation of a hospital, they would only do so if the hospital already had a well known history of avoidable patient deaths, or had experienced other adverse publicity. As with NHS managers and officials, the CQC seem to prefer a *See no evil! Hear no evil!* approach to dealing with problems, and tend to lean to the side that has the power which, of course, is never the employee.

The balance between employers (such as hospitals) and staff (nurses etc) is tilted to favour the employers, who are always in a no lose situation when they punish staff for speaking out about patient safety and related issues, whereas staff are always in a no win situation when they do speak out.

♧ Registration Bodies – Hidden Agenda

Registration bodies are agents who are tasked to protect, promote, and maintain the health and safety of the public and, in this role, they are classified as "prescribed persons", to whom employees can make protected disclosures concerning health and safety and other public interest issues. When whistleblowers make their protected disclosures to those registration bodies, their purpose also has the aim of protecting/promoting the health and safety of patients. It would seem reasonable, therefore, that the registration bodies would encourage employees to help them in meeting their public health and safety objectives, and would support whistleblowers in making their disclosures, and protect them from retribution from employers for making those disclosures.

This is not how the registration bodies behave. Instead, the employers of whistleblowers will call on the registration bodies to inflict punitive actions on the whistleblowers, with justifications manufactured by managers. As a result, whistleblowers might expect suspension or termination of their registrations, and suffer the loss of their livelihoods that accompany such punishments.

What the registration bodies do, effectively, is collude with NHS employers to protect and maintain the NHS cover-up culture, as a priority over protecting and maintaining the health and safety of the public, which is what they exist to do – they are "double agents" of the NHS.

♘ General Medical Council

As an experiment, I wrote to the registration body for doctors, the General Medical Council, and asked what protection they would give to a doctor who may be suffering revenge punishment for raising an issue of public interest (whistleblowing). The answer from the GMC was that doctors are protected from punitive actions by the Public Interest Disclosure Act – the very Act of Parliament that the Francis Report concluded was weak and ineffective, and which the Department of Health has acknowledged is not for purpose. The GMC knows these things, so the only reason they would furnish me with such a dismissive and dishonest answer is because they do NOT provide protection for doctors who speak out about their concerns. What the GMC do is what every other government body does, which is protect the public image of the government by telling me what I think is the right "answer" to my question.

🚜 Motivations for False Accusations

Disciplinary action is cruelly wielded against any employee who does not comply with NHS propaganda or the cover-up culture, usually with fabricated stories of the victim being aggressive to their colleagues. It is impossible for the accused employee to successfully present a winning defensive argument to any accusations made by the employer, because of the absence of natural justice and, for those NHS workers who decide to defend themselves, the only effective strategy they can take, is to go on the offensive, and voice their own counter accusations against the employer. The way to do that is for the employee to learn why they have been chosen for disciplinary action, and that means learning what issue it is that the manager wants to suppress, or in what way the employee is a threat to the management hierarchy. Some example motivations for disciplinary actions include discrimination, the manager wants to promote their friend or loyal vassal, revenge, covering up a healthcare issue, and career blocking. I use the term "career blocking" to describe the technique of creating the fiction that an employee is unsuitable for advancement, because they have a disciplinary history, and have suffered the "give a dog a bad name" propaganda against them, and have a "track record" of trouble making.

Disciplinary Tactics

♨ Pattern of Behaviour

When NHS managers decide to punish an employee, they will often use the trick of establishing a "pattern of behaviour" against them, often in the form of false accusations of bullying, made by the victim's colleagues who, in one way or another, will benefit from helping management in their persecution of the victim. If there is only one accusation, no disciplinary action can be taken, because that would be too easy to counter, at an Employment Tribunal. If, however, three or more people make false accusations against the target of management's ire, the "pattern of behaviour" tactic is used by the personnel department, as "proof" that the victim is guilty of whatever they are accused of, and that allows disciplinary action to be taken, in the form of a warning, dismissal for gross misconduct, or reporting to the victim's registration body (GMC/NMC/HCPC). Regardless of the type of punishment, the victim's career prospects will have been stifled, and that is the deterrent that managers use to prevent other staff from also considering taking whatever actions that might pose a threat to the employer.

During their disciplinary Hearing, the victim is prevented from introducing information regarding motivating factors for the accusations made against them, and is not allowed to include details of how the accusers are rewarded with, for example, promotion, or improved holiday and shift patterns. The personnel clerks will also refuse to allow submission of information of how some of the accusers may be beholding to management, because they are fraudulently qualified, not adequately competent, or are drug users. These people, incidentally, support management and the cover-up culture because they, themselves, depend on it.

The pattern of behaviour accusation is not symmetrically utilised, senior staff can use the technique against junior staff, but junior staff cannot use it against senior staff. An employee cannot, for example, make a formal complaint that they have suffered any form of bullying or intimidation, on multiple occasions, against a senior person, or a peer who is an ally of the senior person.

When management use a "pattern of behaviour" as virtual evidence of a misdeed by an NHS employee, in place of real evidence, it is a sure sign that the case against the employee has been fabricated. This tactic is so frequently used that it is almost comically predictable. As Inspector Clouseau might say: "Aah, yeees! The old pattern of behaviour ploy!".

⚔ Balance of Probability

To make it appear that a disciplinary panel of senior nurses and personnel department clerks have acted in a jurisprudential manner, they will claim that their guilty ruling is based on "the balance of probability", but they do not illustrate how they have measured or balanced the probabilities, or even identified what the probabilities are. The reason for that is that they have not used the balance of probabilities at all, because they do not understand the term any more than they understand the law or human rights. Saying "balance of probability" makes them believe that it convinces others that they have acted with propriety.

⚐ Rewarding the Bullies

After successfully punishing the victim of a manager's harassment, the victim's accusers (bullies) will be rewarded for their loyalty, either by career enhancing steps, such as accelerated promotion, or approval of certain requests, such as leave times, or transfer to preferred work areas. This is how weaker and "ungifted" employees make career progress – not by meritorious work and intelligence, but for subservience and obsequiousness to their autocratic and corrupt superiors.

Psychologists label the practice, by these less able people, of bullying on behalf of their managers, as "over compensation", which means to counter their inadequacies by excelling in other areas. In the NHS, excelling does not mean excellence in service delivery to patients, it means promotion or being rewarded with easy and non-stressful jobs, such as working in simulation centres, becoming *Freedom To Speak Up Guardians*, or working as clinical practice educators. (In fairness, some clinical practice educators do have the right attributes of intelligence, knowledge, and keenness to help others, but these people are rare.)

♨ Disciplinary Case Packs

Another NHS personnel department disciplinary tactic is to overwhelm the accused worker (victim) with large disciplinary document packs, which contain the employer's voluminous Disciplinary Policy, witness statements, and the case document that details the accusations against them. Most victims of disciplinary action are junior clinical staff (band 5/6), such as nurses and anaesthetic technicians, and these people, in the main, are neither well read, nor do they possess any sort of investigative skill which might equip them to analyse their documentary case files. Consequently, upon receipt of a large bundle of disciplinary case documentation, the accused victim will, typically, respond by handing in their notice, or simply submitting to the attacks made on them.

Quitting their jobs is, incidentally, often one of the outcomes which a manager aims for – it is much easier than sacking the employee, then hoping that the employee will not take independent defensive legal action, which would mean civil procedures being conducted in a public forum – which runs contrary to the aims of the NHS cover-up culture. Managers know how easy it is to "stimulate" an employee into taking the route of seeking alternative employment, and they do this on such a frequent basis, that it can be considered normal practice.

♨ Hidden Voice Recordings

One indication of whether or not a hospital's disciplinary Hearing system might be fair and impartial, is their attitude to recording meetings and Hearings. If the hospital has a policy of recording proceedings, and distributing copies of the recordings to all parties, it might well be that their procedures are conducted with propriety or, at least partly so. Alternatively, if no recordings are permitted, it is a clear sign that proceedings will be unfair, the personnel department representative and/or other Hearing members will make their own covert recordings, and official minutes of the Hearing will be inaccurate, and biased against the victim.

St George's Hospital (Tooting) exemplifies this particular dirty trick, because it has a published policy of prohibiting hidden recordings, yet managers and the principle personnel department clerk, Alfred Neuman, responsible for disciplinary cases (case manager), makes hidden voice recordings at disciplinary Hearings, using such devices disguised as pens and phone chargers.

Incidentally, it is not just at formal disciplinary Hearings that these recording gadgets are used; senior staff (mostly) will also use them at informal meetings with the targets of their scheming, and where there are no witnesses present. To ensure that their victim is unprepared to make their own covert audio recording, the manager will arrange it so that the meeting is a spontaneous, rather than a planned event of the "Oh! I'm glad I bumped into you. Have you got a minute?" type.

An employee, after attending one of these informal meetings, should not be surprised when, some considerable time later, the manager is able to recall the contents of the meeting in great detail, and will share confidences with other staff members.

🎤 Evidence

When someone leaves their phone charger or other device plugged in, close to where you (target) work, it is not always because they "forgot it", it might be because the charger contains a voice activated recording device. This is something that I first discovered when I observed a colleague, a cocaine user and partying friend of the anaesthetic team leader leave her phone charger plugged in at my work area (anaesthetic room). When my surgical list finished, I was moved to another operating theatre and, whilst I was busy checking a patient in, that phone charger (same stain on the label), as if by magic, appeared in my new anaesthetic room. Very suspicious! At the earliest opportunity, I marked the charger by using a surgical blade (scalpel) to cut two very small lines into the body of the charger. After work, I searched the internet for covert recording devices, and found one sold by the "Spy Shop" (Oxford St).

Two days later, when the owner of the charger that I marked and I were on the same shift, I identified that same charger again, when it was placed in my work area, a short time after the shift started. A quick comparison with the Spy Shop image revealed that it was, indeed, the same model as was advertised. So, my cocaine snorting colleague was recording my private conversations.

It was because of this discovery that, over the following two years, I became wise to these covert devices and, on two other occasions, I replaced phone chargers, that had been left in my work area, with identical but ordinary chargers, and also found that a travel clock was a covert voice recorder. I discussed this matter with a trustworthy colleague, who was being victimised by a team leader (band 7 nurse) for reporting one of her fellow countrymen for being a danger to patients. Some months later, this colleague was called in to her team leader's office, to be abused and criticised for another made up reason. After she (colleague) sat down, the team leader made an excuse to leave the office for a few minutes. When she returned, she was carrying a phone charger. which she plugged in to a wall socket – without a phone attached. There was no good reason for plugging in the phone charger, by itself, so it must have been a voice recorder – there is no other explanation. Clearly, this senior nurse seemed to think that staff in her team were too stupid to consider that she was using a recording device (against trust policy), but that is not too surprising, because she received her promotion for her loyalty to the bullying manager, Cathy Stirling (dope smoker - now retired).

The lesson I learnt from my and my colleague's experiences was that personal and telephone conversations should always be made in the corridor outside of the department, and away from people and electrical devices, because there is always someone who will want to gather ammunition that can be used against you, in return for sycophantic reward from the interested manager.

♣ Employment Tribunals

When a "targeted" employee considers whether or not to use their own covert recording devices, contrary to their employer's policy, it is worth knowing that the official Employment Tribunal policy that these hidden recordings ARE acceptable for submission as evidence. Submission of such recordings, however, must be accompanied by written transcripts of the recordings, and use of the recordings must be justified, and must not be used with the aim of entrapment or to gain a dishonest advantage.

⚙ Confidentiality

Disciplinary packs include instructions for the victim to refrain from discussing their case with other members of staff. Complying with such an instruction does not benefit the victim, it hinders them, because it prevents them from learning from the experiences of colleagues who have also suffered disciplinary action. It also has the objective of making the employee feel isolated and vulnerable. If management discover that a victim of disciplinary action has discussed their case with a colleague, it becomes extra ammunition to use against them – it adds to a pattern of negative behaviour. Isolation has the added benefit of inflicting psychological damage on the employee and, if the employee is a whistleblower, who poses a threat to the NHS cover-up culture, the persistent and cumulative psychologically damaging effects might even stimulate the employee into committing suicide (it does happen), thereby removing the whistleblowing threat.

Legal Attacks

A hospital's personnel department clerks, with the help of departmental managers (mostly nurses, sometimes doctors), execute disciplinary actions on a daily basis, and the experience they gain from any case helps them in subsequent cases. This advantage of disciplinary experience does not extend to victims of disciplinary action, these people are very much on their own, and most victims drown in such an unfamiliar and hostile environment as a disciplinary Hearing. With such an overwhelming advantage of experience (and dirty tricks), personnel clerks and department managers should be able to conduct their Hearings without outside assistance, but they don't. If a disciplinary victim decides to defend themselves, and takes the issue to an employment tribunal, or civil court, the hospital will allocate large amounts of taxpayer's money (seven or eight figure sums annually) to commission law firms to fight their (the hospital's) case for them. The victim, of course, is not allocated legal counsel; they have to suffer the onslaught of legal experts, and their accompanying legal tricks and booby-traps. Why this happens is clear, by using expert legal help, the hospital is almost guaranteed to win the case against the employee, and this is proof that the disciplinary case is neither fair nor moral.

⚔ Legal Protection for Chief Executives

As an aside to the above issue, it might be of interest to NHS employees and the public alike, to consider the advertising message from one law firm, which specialises in healthcare issues, such as action against employees, and defending NHS executives with their propaganda tricks:

"We also know that reputational stakes are high. The decisions you take may have significant ramifications. We offer timely advice that can prevent career-ending, reputational damage caused by factors ranging from negligence to poor governance."

What they are saying, in a roundabout way, is that if a hospital's Chief Executive is vulnerable to negative press, because of some issue where patients have suffered harm, or is of a fraudulent or corrupt nature, the law firm will manipulate the situation to minimise any bad publicity, and protect the Chief Executive's position. All this, naturally, can be achieved for a generous fee – paid for by the taxpayer. Perhaps some people are more equal than others. (The following chapter expands on some of the above disciplinary process "dirty tricks" used against employees.)

16: DISCIPLINARY DIRTY TRICKS

When a manager wants to "remove", or cause other types of harm, to an employee, particularly a whistleblower, they do so by creating the fiction that the employee is in breach of a legal or professional requirement, or code of conduct, of one type or another. Managers have to do this so that they appear to have justification in taking disciplinary action against the employee, otherwise the disciplinary process would not stand up to scrutiny, should the employee proceed to an Employment Tribunal.

A Disciplinary Hearing is a sham process, that allows management to give the impression that they reach their punishment decisions based on evidence and procedure, proved by their records of the case in question. The case files, themselves, will fraudulently describe how the proceedings were fair, and the members of the Disciplinary Panel were independent and impartial.

To ensure that the Disciplinary Process achieves the outcome that management have already decided for the employee, various "dirty tricks" are used against them, with some of the more common tricks listed below. To personalise the disciplinary experience, the list of dirty tricks are presented (with some duplication) in the form of advice to you, the whistleblowing reader, in the second person, as if you are the one being disciplined.

♣ Dirty Tricks

♠ Impartiality

Disciplinary Panel members are supposed to be impartial and independent, without allegiance or bias, one way or the other. They are, in fact, just the opposite. If management have already decided the outcome of the Hearing, which should always be assumed to be the case, then each Panel member is obliged to concur with whatever that decision is. Anyone who does not do so will be in opposition to the bullying practices of the hospital and, it follows, that they will also be in opposition to the cover-up culture that the hospital relies on for its positive image. The Panel members know that they have to be compliant – because it is that compliance that allows them to keep their senior positions.

♠ Disciplinary Pack

Prior to the Disciplinary Hearing, the case manager (personnel department clerk) will send you your disciplinary pack which, as mentioned in the previous chapter, will contain lots of information. The disproportionately large disciplinary policy is meant to be intimidating, and to make you feel overwhelmed with the amount of information that you have to assimilate. Having to read the policy also serves to reduce the amount of time you will have to read the case document (accusations against you), which means you will have less opportunity to give it a forensic examination and, consequently, you will be less likely to spot the errors and inconsistencies that it will inevitably contain.

❁ Receipt of the Disciplinary Case Document

The disciplinary pack will contain an instruction that you sign one of the copies of the case document, and return it immediately to the case manager. The case document will, almost certainly, be littered with misleading information and fabrications, all designed to make you appear guilty of misconduct. By signing the case document, you will be agreeing with the contents, so DO NOT SIGN IT. There is no benefit to you, the accused employee, in signing for this or any other document you receive, and there is no legal or moral requirement for you to do so – so don't. If the case manager tries to pressure you into signing this or any other document (unless you wrote it), politely tell them that you will not, and ask them to send you, in writing, their reasons for asking you to provide your signature to the documents they send you.

Making you sign for a document, at the very start of the Disciplinary process, is the way that the case manager hopes to instill in you the habit of signing for things so that, when they eventually send you written transcripts of any of your Hearings, you might automatically, through habit, follow the instruction to immediately sign and return the transcript, without firstly scrutinising the contents. What you will be signing for, as already mentioned, is that you agree with the contents of the document, including false information that weakens your defence. So, for emphasis, DO NOT SIGN FOR ANYTHING WRITTEN BY SOMEONE ELSE!

❁ Setting The Hearing Date

The Case Manager will send you the date of the disciplinary Hearing, which will probably be on your day off, and will ask you to confirm, in writing (or email), your agreement to that date. The date of the Hearing will be the earliest convenient date that all Panel members will be available to attend, but there will be no consideration of what is convenient for you, or whether you have enough time to prepare your response document. Indeed, the case manager wants to deny you any advantage, convenience, or feeling that you have any control of the situation. Incidentally, not allowing you the time and opportunity to properly scrutinise the case against you, is a contravention of Article 6 of the Human Rights Act. Do not, therefore, accept the Hearing date that the case manager tries to impose upon you. Instead, provide the case manager a selection of dates that suit you, and your union helper, and that give you enough time to prepare your defence (response) document. Also, do not suggest or accept any Hearing date that falls on one of your days off.

If the case manager takes offence at your affrontery for attempting to set the agenda, and to remove some of the power he (it usually is a "he") has over you, then that is a sure sign that he has no intention of showing you any freedom, courtesy, or generosity, and is not being fair and impartial. If he attempts any sort of intimidation against you, write a letter of complaint about his hostile and bullying behaviour, including the request that he be replaced, then send the letter to the Chief Executive. You have nothing to lose in showing that you will not be manipulated or intimidated; after all, the outcome of the disciplinary process has already been decided, so standing up for yourself will not harm your case.

By making a formal complaint about bullying, you will not only be exercising your human right to be treated with respect and dignity, but you will also frighten the other Panel members into reconsidering the use of some of the dirty tricks they have planned for you. These people are ALL sycophants to the Chief Executive, otherwise they would not have reached their senior positions, and those positions will be weakened if they drag the Chief Executive into a matter that might culminate in the public spectacle that is an Employment Tribunal. Bullies are not brave.

It should also be borne in mind that by weakening the position of the case manager, the other Panel members are less likely to collude with his underhand tricks, because they want to portray themselves as having always acted with propriety, should they be summoned to an Employment Tribunal, or other civil court.

✸ Hearing Date Conflicts

If the case manager refuses to accept a Hearing Date that suits you, he might threaten to hold the Hearing without you. If so, inform him that his decision would be in contravention of Article 6 of the Human Rights Act and, if he proceeds with his threat, inform him also that you will take your case to an Employment Tribunal, and follow that with a complaint to the Health Service Ombudsman, your Member of Parliament, the Justice Minister, the Secretary of State for Health. Involving external bodies is something that weakens the "cover-up" ethos of the employer, who will not, on the whole, expect an employee to have the fortitude to make complaints to external bodies, so they are unlikely to dismiss what you say as bluff.

Disciplinary panel members are lower and middle management only and, if they want to proceed to higher management, they have to maintain the cover-up culture, by keeping issues in-house. They wll, therefore, do an about turn and do their best to satisfy your suggestions for Hearing dates. If not, then do not cave in and attend the Hearing on a date that is not suitable for you. Let the Panel conduct the Hearing without you, after all, the outcome will be no different than if you were present.

❋ Hearing Date On Your Day Off

As mentioned above, do not be surprised if the case manager tries to force you (target) to accept a Hearing date on your day off. That is another way of exercising power, and making you feel like there is no escape from the their tyranny. None of the panel members will attend the Hearing on their days off, so neither should you.

If, after the panel have acquiesced to your insistence that the Hearing not take place on your day off, and they have accepted one of your own preferred dates, you might discover that your manager (or team leader) changes your shift roster, without informing you, so that the revised roster lists a day off coinciding with your new Hearing date. In such an instance, the first thing to do is make a copy of the revised roster, so that you have proof of the changes the manager has made. Do not let your manager know that you have noticed the changes to your roster, and do not inform the Hearing panel of those changes, until you are as close to the Hearing date as possible. Then, inform the case manager that you have only just discovered the underhand trick played on you, that you are disgusted by what has happened, and you regard it as another example of bullying. Also tell the case manager that you will not, under any circumstances, attend a Hearing on one of your days off, and provide him with other dates that are convenient to you.

Do not try to resolve the problem of your roster changes yourself –

leave that problem to others. (It won't take long for the case manager to undo the changes that your manager made to your roster.)

⊛ Sending your Response Document

After you have agreed a convenient (to you) Hearing date, the case manager will ask you to send in your written response to the accusations against you. He will want to receive that document well before the Hearing date, so that the whole Panel will have plenty of time to familiarise themselves with your defence, and will have time to prepare any dirty tricks that will undermine you. Do not send in your response document until as close to the Hearing date as possible, so that you give the Panel the same disadvantage of limited time that they tried to impose on you. If, by doing so, the panel decide that they do not have enough time to read your response document, offer them a choice of other Hearing dates. Do not think that being kind or helpful to the Panel will produce any sort of fairness or propriety in them – it will not change their agenda, which is to harm you.

⊛ Relevant Information

To limit your ability to defend against the accusations made against you, the case manager will inform you that the Panel will not accept information that does not directly concern those accusations. The Panel will not, for example, accept your argument that you are being punished for raising issues about fraud or patient safety, you are being discriminated against, or because the manager wants to clear you from the path to promoting a favourite employee, who is less deserving than you of the promotion.

You cannot stop the Panel from disregarding the real reasons why you are being punished, but neither can the Panel stop you from including this information in your written defence - your response document – and they cannot stop you from insisting on focusing on the motivations at your Hearing. When the Hearing Manager realises that the Panel are starting to lose control of events, because you are discussing the truth and motivations about your case, he may threaten to abandon the Hearing, if you do not stick to the Panel's agenda. Respond by informing the Panel that you have a legal right to present your defence with any information that you deem pertinent to the accusations made against you.

It should be borne in mind that, just because the case manager makes prohibitions about what you are or are not allowed to present in your attempts to defend yourself, there is no legal obligation for you to comply with his directives. You have every right to act within the constraints of what the law allows, and not by your employer's diktats. You should, therefore, not hesitate to complain, in WRITING, about any restriction that weakens your ability to present your case.

If the Panel abandon the Hearing, make a WRITTEN complaint, to the Personal Department Director (cc to the Chief Executive), about how the Panel halted the Hearing because they could not fight against the truth that you were confronting them with.

⚘ Seating

When arriving at the Disciplinary Hearing venue, the Panel will probably already be seated, and will be situated in such a way that is most advantageous to them by, for example, ensuring that the remaining seats are close to their surreptitiously placed audio recording devices. If the room has a window, and has a sunny aspect, the available seats face into the sun, so that you are "blinded" by the light, and that will be uncomfortable and distracting for you.

At one hospital, a union representative warned a paramedic of these tactics. When they arrived at the Hearing venue - a small conference room – the two available seats were facing the sun, as the union rep predicted, and there was a phone charger plugged into a wall socket, immediately behind the empty seats. Before sitting down, the paramedic bent towards the phone charger, and chanted "1-2, 1-2. Testing! Testing!", then sat down and donned his sunglasses. None of the Panel members commented on his "Testing" for volume level, but the case manager asked him to remove his sunglasses. The paramedic announced "Facing into the sun would permanently damage my eyes. You have put me in a position of harm, and you have failed to provide me with Personal Protective Equipment (PPE), which is a criminal offence. I have had to supply my own PPE. Do you want to repeat your instruction?" The case manager was, apparently, so stunned by this turn of events, that he failed to reply. Needless to say, no more was said by anyone about the matter and, according to the union rep, none of the Panel members made any of the accusatory and aggressive attacks that usually accompany the Hearing process. (Two weeks later, sun blinds were fitted to the window.)

This issue of being proactive against Disciplinary Panel dirty tricks may seem trivial, but it does put Panel members on their guard, weakens their resolve, reduces their confidence, and inflicts on them the same psychological assault that they try to inflict on their victims. Small victories can have an accumulative effect.

✸ Hidden Recordings

To emphasise the importance of being aware of Disciplinary Panels making covert recordings, it should always be assumed that covert recordings will be made at any Hearing or informal meeting you have with managers and personnel department clerks. If you do not also make a covert recording of any Hearing or private meeting, you will have no proof (for an Employment Tribunal) that transcripts from case managers are inaccurate records of what was really said, or by whom. You will see the value of making your own covert recording when you receive the Panel's transcript (disguised as meeting "minutes") of your Hearing, because it will be inaccurate, misleading, and biased against you. An audio recording provides proof of the discrepancies that the transcript will contain.

If your employer discovers that you have made hidden recordings, further disciplinary action might be made against you, so you should only make recordings if you are certain that you are going to take your case to an Employment Tribunal, and are confident that you have valid reasons for making those recordings.

✸ Yes or No?

A recurring tactic of Disciplinary Panel members, and other inquisitors, is to try to force you to give a "yes" or "no" answer to a question, when "yes" or "no" are not appropriate answers to that question. In such an event, inform the questionner that you will listen to any question posed, but you will choose in what way you will answer the question and, indeed, whether or not you will answer the question at all. That is your right.

✹ Go On The Attack – Present Your Position

Remember that it is not possible to successfully defend yourself at an NHS Disciplinary Hearing – the outcome is pre-decided - but you do have to go through the motions of the Hearing processes, otherwise an Employment Tribunal will refuse to accept your case, because you have not made all reasonable attempts to gain redress. Remember, also, that you should not restrict yourself to defence only, you should go on the attack – make written complaints about every lie, inaccuracy, and disadvantage the process has forced on you. If you do not disagree or complain about something, in WRITING, you are assumed to be in agreement with it. You have a right to complain, so do not hesitate to do so.

Also - to repeat what has previously been mentioned - just because the case manager has prohibited you from including information that he regards as not being directly related to the accusations against you, stick to your guns, and repeatedly raise the issue of being punished for the motivations of your accusers, whether it be because you have raised issues of concern, or for other reasons of hostility against you. The agenda should be set by the underlying reasons for punishing you, and should include mention of who it is that will benefit from disciplinary action against you, and in what way they will benefit.

✹ Returning a Signed Transcript

Some days after the Hearing, you will receive a transcript of the meeting, along with an instruction to return a signed copy as soon as possible. If you do return a signed copy of the transcript, you will be affirming your agreement with the contents. The transcript will not be accurate or fair, so DO NOT SIGN THE TRANSCRIPT.

✸ Appeal Hearing and Employment Tribunal

Once you receive the Hearing's ruling about your guilt, request an Appeal Hearing then, after the Appeal fails, proceed down the route of an Employment Tribunal, and demonstrate to the Tribunal the real reasons and motivations for the case being made against you. Also, of course, present your list of the tricks and unfair practices that your employer has used to weaken your defence.

✸ Punish to Demoralise

To be found guilty at a Disciplinary Process is how management punish you for failing to conform to the sycophantic, cover-up, and conniving NHS work model. Additionally, being found guilty of an offence produces a halt to your career progression – it prevents you from reaching your full career potential. Those who do comply with the malicious and self-serving NHS culture do not ever suffer disciplinary actions, regardless of what harm they do to patients; their loyalty to, and protection of, the NHS bourgeoisie (ruling elite) gives them career security, and allows professional advancement, so that they join and strengthen the management clan.

The effect of disciplinary action is life changing, and will inflict on you, the whistleblower, a psychological blow that is impossible to recover from. What makes the disciplinary and punishment experience most difficult to come to terms with is the fact that, for being a whistleblower, you have been harmed for acting in the interests of patients, for complying with your legal and professional requirements, for doing what the public expect of you and for complying with the general medical mantra of "do no harm".

The cumulative effect of these feelings and realisations is a psychological assault that will make you vulnerable to depression, feelings of isolation, and mental and other health problems. The NHS are aware of these things, and that is why managers like to use the formal disciplinary process against whistleblowers, or anyone else who might be a threat to the positive image of the NHS – they know how victims will suffer, and they know that some of those victims will be so crushed by their disciplinary experiences, that they will consider suicide as their only release from the depression that the NHS has inflicted on them.

The disciplinary process, for some employees, is a virtual firing squad, and nobody in the NHS, or government, cares about that.

✺ Employment Tribunal

When an employee decides to take their employer to an Employment Tribunal, typically because of bullying, managers will often nullify the possibility of facing the Tribunal, by using tactics such as promising to look for another job that the employee can transfer to, and where they will not have to work alongside those who have bullied them. In their new job, the employee will be properly treated, until 3 months have passed since the start of their complaint. After that time, the employee does not have the option of an Employment Tribunal, because there is a maximum of 3 months allowed between the initial complaint, and lodgement of a claim with the Tribunal Service. It is an often used trick against employees.

Final Advice

The final thing to remember about disciplinary Hearings, is that you should be calm throughout. If you get emotional, or angry, you will look weak, and will be vulnerable to accusations of being aggressive or unstable (*tone policing*). You should also remember that you can only fight your case with what you WRITE – not what you say.

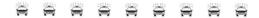

⛟ 17: DRUG ADDICTED STAFF

According to the *International Nurses Society on Addictions*, "Substance abuse is a serious problem in the medical profession, and it places patients at risk of injury or death."

For NHS patients, the risk of serious injury or death should be of particular concern because, according to the *European Monitoring Centre for Drugs and Drug Addiction (EMCDDA)*, Great Britain is the drugs capital of Europe, with higher levels of cocaine, cannabis, and amphetamine abuse than anywhere else in Europe. The delivery of safe and effective healthcare services cannot be guaranteed, if the person delivering the care is working under the residual influence of drugs, so this is an issue that must be removed from the protective umbrella of the NHS cover-up culture, if patients are to be kept safe from the administration of care services from drug users.

According to the EMCDDA, one in four adults in London, at weekends, takes cocaine, so, the probability that NHS clinical staff (nurses, doctors, anaesthetic technicians) are **not** drug users is too small to be considered realistic. One in four clinical professionals therefore, must be considered to be regular drug users and, by inference, one in four of those people pose a risk to patients.

To combat the dangers caused by staff working under the influence of drugs, the UK Health and Safety Executive (HSE) give instructions on how employers should mitigate against those dangers, and explains how failing to do so contravenes the Health and Safety at Work Act, which is a criminal offence.

The NHS, however, does not acknowledge that drug use is a problem amongst employees, does not follow HSE guidelines on managing drug abuse, and does not employ any system of screening, either as part of initial training and recruitment schemes, or as part of ongoing and proactive safety assessments. This is even though NHS officials know that drug abuse permeates all levels of British society, including the Houses of Commons and Lords - there is no secret about that. This being the case, why does the NHS not acknowledge that drug abuse, by clinical staff, poses a potential risk to patients? Are they covering it up? Apparently so.

It is only when an NHS employee receives a criminal prosecution for drug offences that the hospital, or other NHS employer, dismisses the employee, not because their drug use poses a risk to patient safety, but because of the bad publicity which could ensue, should patients discover that the hospital employs such addicts. In the NHS, a positive image is everything, and no news is good news, so preventing bad news concerning patient safety from reaching the public is given higher priority than addressing the safety risk posed by drug using clinical staff.

⚘ Precautionary Principle

In terms of safety, it would be prudent for the NHS to comply with the *Precautionary Principle*, and assume that, until proved otherwise, all hospital staff involved in clinical care are active drug users and, as such, are a constant threat to patient safety. At the very least, the NHS should assume that the number of drug using staff matches the EMCDDA one in four figure and, with some urgency, should create systems to filter out those drug users.

Being precautionary is the safe attitude to take, but this is the attitude which the NHS avoids, because it would adversely affect targets for staffing levels and, more significantly, its public image, and that, of course, contravenes the NHS cover-up culture.

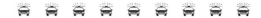

⛟ 18: DRUG ADDICT COVER-UP

There are many doctors, nurses, health care assistants, paramedics, and operating department practitioners who are habitual and addicted users of cocaine, cannabis, crack, heroin, and benzodiazepines, and they all pose a hazard to patient safety, because their otherwise normal behaviours and thought patterns are modified by the drugs they use. NHS officials prefer to take a "hear no evil, see no evil" approach to drug abuse by staff, and it is this instinct to cover-up the problem that protects these drug users.

One telling account of how a drug user has been protected by the NHS cover-up culture, in an attempt to minimise the publicity of the account, concerns that of a senior anaesthetic technician (Operating Department Practitioner) at St George's Hospital, in Tooting. This anaesthetic technician used to steal pain-relieving drugs, meant for surgical patients, and replace them with syringes containing normal saline solution. (He was also thought to have spiked the fake syringes with beta blocking agents, to simulate the effects of analgesia.) The consequence of a surgical patient not receiving their pain relieving drugs can lead to extreme harm, including cardiac arrest and death, so this is a safety critical matter.

As a heroin addict, the technician found it irresistable to steal pharmacological diamorphine, the *British Approved Name* for heroin, from the maternity unit. (Diamorphine is what is given to mothers who undergo Caesarian Section procedures.)

To disguise his drug thefts, which went on for several years, the technician recorded issuance of drugs to so called "ghost" patients, in the controlled drugs register, and reported other ampoules that he stole as being dropped and broken. There was so much repetition of these accounts of drug "waste" that the Operating Theatre Department were unable to keep this issue internal to the department, because the pharmacy department decided that evidence of drug thefts was too clear to be ignored, and so they commenced formal investigations into the thefts. To hide evidence of his thefts, the anaesthetic technician stole and disposed of the controlled drug registers. Consequently, because stealing drug registers is a criminal offence, the hospital could not avoid reporting the matter to the police, and the anaesthetic technician was suspended. The hospital had no choice but to report him to his registration body, the Health and Care Professions Council (HCPC).

At his HCPC disciplinary Hearing, the anaesthetic technician was accompanied by an anaesthetist, Dr Hampson-Evans, who is employed by St George's hospital (Tooting), and works on his days off at Princess Grace hospital (London). Dr Hampson-Evans defended the technician, and assured the HCPC that the technician was determined to end his drug habit. According to Dr Hampson-Evans, this was an exemplary practitioner, who was "better inside the system than outside".

Because of this testimony, the HCPC decided to be generous and, instead of removing the technician's registration, they suspended it for one year. By convincing the HCPC that the technician was an asset to the NHS, and was committed to ending his drug habit, Dr Hampson-Evans minimised any adverse publicity against the hospital (a suspension is not as news-worthy as a striking off order).

After his suspension, the anaesthetic technician found employment at Kingston Hospital, where he resumed his drug stealing almost from the first day in his new job. It took the hospital less than six weeks to conclusively determine that he was stealing drugs and, after involvement of the police, he was dismissed, and the HCPC removed his registration – this time, permanently.

One distinguishing characteristic of this case concerns that of Dr Hampson-Evans, whose defence and salutations of the anaesthetic technician allowed him (technician) to resume his career, and to continue his theft and use of drugs. This was very strange behaviour for a doctor because, as a rule, doctors do NOT give testimonial support to drug addicted staff – it didn't happen before this case, and it hasn't happened since.

Notably, neither the above account of a drug addicted clinical professional, nor any of the other employees caught stealing or using drugs, convinced St. George's Hospital to initiate a drug screening regime, because that would have conflicted with the hospital's cover-up culture, and put the chief executive's position at risk.

⛬ 19: FAKE QUALIFICATIONS

The work of nurses and anaesthetic technicians was, originally, based on supporting surgeons and anaesthetists in executing the practical aspects of healthcare delivery. These nursing and technician roles were semi-skilled, required positive personal characteristics, such as common sense, industry, practicality, honesty, cleanliness, and a caring attitude towards patients, but did not require much more than a basic education. For doctors, the situation is different, because there is a direct correlation between education and efficacy of patient care, so they have to be well educated to be able to understand the causes and cures of disease conditions.

⛬ Nurses and Allied Professionals

In recent decades, nurses and anaesthetic technicians (and other allied health trades) have evolved into what the NHS describes as autonomous professionals, whose members are qualified to degree level (Bachelor of Science), and who take part, in theory, in the assessment, diagnosis, and treatment of patients. To reflect this change in professional roles, the official job title of the anaesthetic technician has been changed from its original name of *Operating Department Assistant*, to that of *Operating Department*

Practitioner, and the educational qualification has changed from an unrecognised diploma to a Bachelor of Science degree. Similarly, the old junior role of "enrolled" nurse has disappeared, and all nurses are now B.Sc. degree educated "registered" nurses.

Given the above educational criteria for nurses and anaesthetic technicians, it would be reasonable to assume that these people have science degree level knowledge, and do make autonomous decisions about the delivery of healthcare services to patients. This is not so. Nurses and anaesthetic technicians, with very few exceptions, work as they always have done; they follow instructions from doctors, and do not take part in anything other than trivial decision making processes for patient care. The basic educational and intelligence aspects of these two roles is also unchanged from the earlier model (not much different from Victorian times); the only difference is that someone who qualified as a nurse in, say, 1970, might have left school with no significant qualifications, as opposed to someone qualifying with a Bachelor of Science degree in nursing or Operating Department Practice today who, typically, left school with a bucketful of GCSE qualifications of the "media studies" and "sociology" ilk, but with the same intelligence and knowledge level of the 1970's person, with virtually no knowledge of science, and without even the most basic numeracy and literacy skills (there are exceptions).

This fact is easy to demonstrate, by simple inquisition of knowledge levels for nurse and anaesthetic technician (ODP) graduates. As an example of the deficiency in science knowledge for these nurses and technicians, it is almost always the case that most of them do not understand even the most basic concepts of science (SI units, percentages, ratios, pressure, force, density, gradients, osmosis, diffusion, arithmetic, atomic structure, the periodic table, ...). A memorable example of how fraudulent these healthcare degrees are, concerns that of a senior midwife (B.Sc.) in charge of a shift, who asked a paediatric doctor if *covalent bonding* had something to do with mother and baby when, in fact, it is a chemical process.

What is also commonly the case is lack of basic literacy skills, such as capitalisation, clauses, punctuation, sentence construction, and the components necessary to make a coherent sentence. These matters of education are at the junior high school level, and form the most basic starting points for eventual study of university science courses, but they are absent in many of these healthcare science graduates.

How it is possible for a science graduate, from a British university (e.g. South Bank), to not have the most basic understanding of the building blocks of scientific study, what our American cousins would refer to as "Science 101"? Such a lack is a shocking indictment of modern British education, and reflects the overall propaganda concerning the benefits of university qualifications for "everyone". What is also shocking is the fact that many of the most senior and experienced nurse and anaesthetic technician Clinical Practice Educators (band seven/eight), who are responsible for ensuring that NHS clinical staff meet their registration requirements with respect to knowledge and understanding of medical issues, are not, themselves, educated to a state which might be described as much more than that of primary school level – even when those people have healthcare Master's degree qualifications, but without the commensurate knowledge and intelligence which such qualifications entail. What, then, is the reason for changing nursing (and anaesthetic technician, Paramedic, etc.) from the model of non-academic trade to university graduate profession? The answer to that question is four fold:

● Firstly, by awarding nurses (etc) with science degrees, it raises their status from working class (USA "blue collar") to that of middle class, and that is something which is a significant advantage in British society – nobody wants to be part of the proletariat (the plebs), and this is what helps attract many working class people to the role – they think it is an easy way up the class ladder.

● Secondly, by awarding nursing students with science degrees, it gives justification to making the students pay for their courses. Few people would put themselves into debt for a simple certificate or diploma qualification, so the degree is a sort of bribery, making students think they have joined the elite members of society – the league of university graduates.

● Thirdly, raising the qualification "level" projects a more positive image for the public, because of the implied, but false, corresponding rise in the intelligence level of the nurses and ODPs, so that an implied improvement in care quality is made.

● The fourth factor is that of scapegoating; if an incident occurs where a patient suffers harm, it would be much more reasonable to pass the blame on to nurses who have university degrees, than it would be if nurses were not educated to such a level.

📖 📖 📖 📖 📖

If the introduction of degree qualifications was, indeed, intended to raise intelligence and knowledge levels of the healthcare workforce, then it would be necessary to attract more academically gifted people, and that would only be possible if the remuneration levels were also increased, and if the NHS became a workplace which respected the concepts of staff equality, meritocracy, and quality of care which, currently, is not the case.

Nurse (and allied profession) training does not warrant a university degree, genuine or otherwise, and should not be subject to training fees, by students, unless training is commensurate with high salaries. The better salaries would serve to lessen the financial burden of such training, and make nursing a much more appealing vocation. Assuming that it is extremely unlikely that a British government, of any party, would sanction high pay for nurses (British politicians do not like to see the "oiks" do well), then the only viable option is to make nurse training free of course fees. That would be fair and reasonable, and would help reduce the practice of raiding third world countries of their nursing staff.

🞂 Mentor Qualification

One of the most financially wasteful components of a hospital's training budget, is the allocation of fees to clinical staff who want to attain the so called "Mentor" qualification, which is provided by some universities. The mentor qualification is a prerequisite for anyone who wants to advance beyond the lowest nursing level of band five and, therefore, is a sought after qualification.

The mentorship course, at £1,200 per person, is a short part-time and self-directed learning scheme, is of a very low academic standard, and is very difficult to fail. Mentorship training is a typical NHS style tick box exercise, which helps project the false idea that clinical training is conducted by properly qualified staff and, in so doing, the quality and safety of healthcare delivery is of an assured higher professional standard, than it would otherwise be. The truth is, when someone achieves the mentorship qualification, their ability to do their job, and ability to teach students and junior staff, is no different from before they had the qualification.

Here is the description of mentoring training from NHS England...

"NHS England is committed to creating the culture and conditions for all employees to reach their potential and make the best contribution to improving outcomes for patients. To achieve this we have developed a range of development and support offerings for staff, one of which is mentoring. Mentoring is a central component of NHS England's drive to create, sustain and develop a diverse workforce, where mentors act as role models, and where employees maximise their potential, and their contribution to delivery of healthcare services."

The reality is that mentorship training is just one of the many components of the (false) professional and pro-education image which the NHS wants to paint for itself. It is self serving propaganda, and a waste of taxpayer's money.

⚔ Healthcare Masters Degrees

Another propaganda scam, and waste of taxpayer's money, is that of Master's degree courses in healthcare and healthcare management subjects. These advanced (supposedly) courses do not reflect or deserve their high status as Master's degrees, and they are, at approximately £12,000 a time, not much more than money making schemes for the universities who offer them; these courses are difficult to fail, so they are very popular with staff who seek promotion, especially up to band eight level.

As an example of the weak academic content of these healthcare Master's degree courses, Kingston University offer a Master of Science degree in Clinical Leadership, whose primary content includes the promise to gain practical skills in "advanced decision making, creative problem solving, and critical thinking".

Advanced decision making means looking at information before making the decision.

Creative problem solving means considering more than one option to find a solution to a problem.

Critical thinking is making an objective decision based on facts.

What these three issues mean, for NHS managers, is that they should pause to think before making decisions. (This is not much different from what parents tell children.) It is not, as they say, "rocket science".

For a manager, these qualifications are used as a mechanism to justify promoting a favourite colleague ahead of more deserving candidates. Evidence of that is in the way these courses are allocated; there is no departmental advertising of the fact that a course is available, and no system for allowing competition between staff, or even an opportunity for staff to make an applications for the courses. Managers will allocate courses to the people who they want to promote, then, once those favoured people have completed their courses, they will be seen as the most qualified to take up more senior positions, and will have no competitors for promotion. The NHS is not a meritocracy and, as with everything else written here, the evidence of these fake qualifications is there for anyone to see, if they care to look.

🚑 Immediate Life Support

Clinically registered professionals, such as nurses and anaesthetic technicians, must, as part of their employment and registration, complete biennial Immediate Life Support (ILS) training and assessment. ILS is the "in-hospital" version of the Resuscitation Council's protocol for dealing with victims of cardiac arrest, and is a subject in which every healthcare professional has to be proficient.

The people who deliver ILS training are experienced and capable professionals, mostly emergency care nurses, and they are commissioned to ensure that all staff complete their training and assessments. Delivering these training courses is straight forward, but these instructors do face a political problem, because they have to record every staff member as having passed their ILS competency tests, even though some employees may be hopelessly incompetent. If anyone is deemed to fail their ILS training, that person is unable to continue in their clinical role, which causes an effective reduction in staff numbers, and that compromises safe staffing levels, which is one of the government's reportable "targets". Because of this political issue of safe staff level targets, ILS trainers are not allowed (unofficially) to class any ILS course attendee as having failed (unless an extreme situation), regardless of whether or not the attendee is, themselves, a liability to patient safety.

By recording the false fact that all clinical staff are competent at responding to cardiac arrests, hospital management can make the claim that they are not accountable, should an incompetent but ILS qualified staff member fail to take the necessary steps which might prevent the death of a cardiac arrest victim. It is the falsely qualified ILS employee who will be held accountable, not the hospital, and that is characteristic of NHS strategy – cover up and assign blame.

❦ Workplace Cardiac Arrest Reponse

In addition to the lack of technical competency of some clinical staff, with respect to performing the cardiac arrest algorithm, there is also the problem of staff not properly responding to cardiac arrest events. In some areas, particularly operating theatres, ICU, and emergency departments, response and execution of life support is usually done quite well, and that is down to the fact these areas always have a supply of anaesthetists, who are the experts at dealing with cardiac arrests. These areas also have, usually, nurses who are of a higher level of professionalism, and are used to dealing wth emergencies.

In other areas, the response of some nurses is much less competent. Some will become panic stricken, others will not understand how they should they react and, incredibly, some will not know where the cardiac arrest trolleys are stored.

Fake Nurses

The shortage of nurses and allied professionals is a long standing problem for the NHS, and one caused by the NHS itself. Staff have to do a dirty job, work unsocial hours, are poorly paid, and are not treated with any reasonable degree of dignity or respect. To make matters worse, staff have to function in a system that is plagued by bullying, favouritism, discrimination, fraud, and forced compliance with the NHS cover-up culture.

The problem of staff shortages, for the government, is politically sensitive and, because of that, it is subject to much propaganda; a standing government will make public statements about how they are effectively addressing staff shortages, and opposition parties will attack the government for its failure to ensure safe staffing levels – it is an ongoing soap box drama.

Something that politicians NEVER discuss is the problem of ensuring that clinical workers are properly competent, and have valid qualifications that accurately reflect their abilities, and that is because quality control is not a valued concept for consideration by politicians; moreover, there are no "targets" for qualification validity. It is for this reason that the NHS has no reluctance in dumbing down nursing and allied professions, by employing healthcare assistants who undergo professional sounding, but very shallow, advanced *Nurse Associate* style training, to do most of the jobs that nurses do.

⚜ Fake Qualifications

The lack of scrutiny for job applicant ability and qualifications makes the NHS a magnet for staff from countries where corruption is normal, and purchasing nursing qualification certificates is standard practice. As an example of how easy it is, in some countries, to buy a health profession qualification, the World Health Organisation, in 2016, reported that 57% of doctors, in India, had fraudulent qualifications. If fake doctors are so prevalent, in just one country, it is reasonable to assume that a similar problem exists in other countries, and not only with doctors, there is also an issue with fake nurses. The NHS recruits these fake professionals on an ongoing basis, and some of them do stand out, because they clearly do not understand their jobs but, because they make up the numbers, the government are satisfied. (*British Government* aka "Targets R Us"!)

Fake qualifications can be bought from online companies, such as **https://www.fastDiplomaOnline.com/**, but an even bigger problem is that of fake scrutiny by interviewers, who will disregard checking of ability and qualifications of job applicants who are favoured by the interviewer - a doctor or senior nurse. Knowledgeable NHS staff often discuss these appointments, and the reasons for giving jobs to unsuitable people, which are usually financial reward (back-handers), sexual favours, family, nationality, religious, or racial bias. A similar problem is that of staff with genuine qualifications, but from countries where bribery is used to pass courses, and good references are routinely purchased.

♣ Recto University

An infamous place for fake qualifications is in the Phillippines: Claro M Recto Avenue, Manilla, where forgers openly produce university degrees, driver licences, airline pilot licences, doctor qualifications, passports, and any other type of fake identification that customer's ask for. Jokingly, Recto Avenue is known as "Recto University". This is where many Filipinoes obtain their nursing qualifications, specifically to allow them to then find jobs in other countries, including the UK. How do they pass scrutiny for jobs in the NHS?

There are many ways: they may work for a year or so in a Phillippines hospital, usually as a healthcare assistant, giving them basic familiarity with the job. Their interviewer may be a friend or relative, or might demand a bribe (normal 3rd world behaviour) to gain the job. Additionally, the British government do not insist on thorough scrutiny of applicants, because their priority is satisfying their own targets for staff numbers – to please voters – and employing incompetent or fraudulently qualified staff ensures compliance with the cover-up culture, because fake nurses depend on that culture themselves.

An example of the above practices can be found at St George's Hospital, Tooting, where a nurse successfully "passed" a telephone interview, from Manilla, to gain employment with the hospital's Theatres Department, with no qualification scrutiny, in 1985. This nurse, Luz Villar, used personal relationships with managers to rise to become a matron, and was infamous for bullying nurses who senior staff did not like, or who spoke out about patient safety issues. She was, in fact, an enforcer of the cover-up culture, and was given freedom to bring in family members and friends from the Phillippines, and give them jobs in Theatres, where most of them worked in the Cardiac and Neurosurgery Wing. It is no coincidence that few English staff were employed in that Wing, because the Filipinoes saw them as a threat, should they discover their fake qualifications, inability to safely communicate in English, or perform necessary drug dosage calculations, as required by nursing registration mandates. (Anti-English discrimination is never discussed, in the NHS, but it is very obvious in all London hospitals, particularly at UCLH, Royal Free, Northwick Park, and St George's, because English staff have the ability to recognise fraudulent nurses, so denying them employment helps conceal the fruds.)

In 2019, whilst working in the Day Surgery Unit, police arrested Villar, and she was subsequently charged with illegal money lending, money laundering, and people trafficking. She was sacked some months later, but the hospital refused to make their own investigations about her conduct, because they did not want to attract attention from the press (cover-up culture).

I made a Freedom of Information request of the Nursing and Midwifery Council, about Villar's qualifications, and was informed that she had never been registered with them, confirming that she was working illegally as a nurse. I passed this information on to the CQC, and they informed me that they did not have the power to take action against St George's, and so they would not take the matter further, even though they knew that there was a high likelihood that the remaining Filipino nurses posed a risk to patient safety.

In January 2020, the Theatre Department manager (matron) was sacked, as a result of my complaints about various other corruption issues, and she was replaced by a Filipino nurse, a friend of matron Villar, who immediately strengthened his position by promoting other Filipinoes to senior (band 7/8) roles, and took over the nursing recruitment process from team leaders, who are the people who more normally do the recruiting, so that he could minimise employment of British nurses and Anaesthetic Technicians (ODPs), and keep their numbers just above the level where discrimination would be too obvious to deny, and then only to employ the least experienced and least competent British staff, so that they do not outshine his Filipino community. Of course, the hospital would never admit to anti-English or anti-British discrimination. Instead, the official reasons for employing so many foreign staff, as usual, would be that British people are lazy, they don't want to train as nurses so are in short supply, and foreign staff are better workers. In reality, British staff are unwelcome, because they are a threat to the NHS cover-up culture, whereas third world staff can be depended upon to never raise issues, or proceed down the official whistleblowing route.

In summary: covering up fraud and avoidable harm protects the NHS and government, cover-ups are only possible if staff go along with those cover-ups, and the staff who can be most depended on to cover up issues have something about themselves that they need covering up, and fraudulent qualifications serve that requirement.

⚙ Healthcare Assistants

NHS hospitals are increasingly addressing their staff shortage problems by "training" healthcare assistants to do the work of nurses and anaesthetic technicians. They do this by enrolling a healthcare assistant, with one year of experience, on a short course, after which, they are deemed to be "qualified", effectively, as a junior nurse or anaesthetic technician. The training for these (fake) qualifiers involves attending ten days at university, then undergoing practical experience by shadowing a properly qualified practitioner, such as a nurse, for a period of eight weeks.

There are three course options:

‣ General Practice Nursing

‣ Operating Theatre Practice

‣ Anaesthetic Practice

The cost of attending the ten days at university is £1,700, payable by the taxpayer, and the trainee remains on full pay throughout, giving a total cost, including the eight weeks of shadowing a qualified person, of approximately £6,000.

If using healthcare assistants to replace traditionally qualified staff is to become accepted practice, then it must also be considered a **safe** practice. If so, then why do nurses and anaesthetic technicians have to spend large amounts of money, and apply themselves to three years of training, when they can bypass the process by working as healthcare assistants for twelve months, then enrolling on the above three month scheme, at no cost to themselves? Also, why don't hospitals avoid the problem of nurse shortages by exclusively recruiting uneducated and unqualified people to work as healthcare assistants, and putting them through the above short-cut courses? Is it because hospitals know that these fast track qualifications are not safe, and they continue to also employ properly qualified staff to compensate for the shortcomings of their fake "practitioners"? What about insurance indemnity? If something goes wrong with patient care, is the hospital's insurance policy valid, when some of the people involved in a patient's case are "fake" practitioners?

The answer to these questions is that hospitals dilute the workforce of qualified staff with healthcare assistant fake nurses and anaesthetic technicians, just enough to escape scrutiny. Scrutiny, however, cannot be escaped if a fake practitioner is involved with a patient death, because an official Coroner's Hearing should reveal the use of fake practitioners in the dead patient's case. The hospital, consequently, will have to justify how the use of faux practitioners meets the requirements of the Precautionary Principle, the Health and Safety at Work Act duty to minimise risk, and the expectations of patients and their families. Another question that must be asked is: are insurance companies aware of the use of fake nurses and anaesthetic practitioners in NHS hospitals? If they are, then how does such usage affect the hospital's insurance premiums? This is an important matter of public interest because, if premiums are higher, due to the higher risk of using staff who are not properly qualified, then that extra money has to be diverted away from patient care.

In addition to the safety implications of using fake practitioners, it is also important to consider the problem of what protection these fake practitioner healthcare assistants have from criminal prosecution, should they find themselves as scapegoats for adverse patient outcomes. The blame and scapegoating character of the NHS does not follow the proper format of responsibility being aligned with seniority; in the NHS, blame flows down the chain of command, to the most junior person which, in this case, is the healthcare assistant "practitioner", or *Nurse Associate*. Perhaps planners have thought of this potential problem, and have decided that responsibility for the fake practitioners is passed to qualified supervising nurses and technicians. (More stress for them!)

Employing fake practitioners is a subject that many nurses and anaesthetic practitioners are unhappy about, but are too afraid to question, because they know how their livelihoods will be adversely affected for raising this, or any other issue of public interest, so, predictably, this is another problem that, given time, will only rear its ugly head in a patient safety related incident.

Nurse Associates

To further embed the issue of officially establishing fake nurses into the NHS, the government are attempting to cover-up their fakery by proceeding to wrap the title of "Nurse Associate" around this scheme of unqualified nurses, in an attempt to disguise the lack of credibility that they really have, and made worse by making space for such "Associates" in the rolls of the *Nursing and Midwifery Council,* thereby providing the necessary image of proper structure and professional credibility that are meant to assure the public.

English Language Skills

In any environment such as healthcare, where the ability to communicate in English is an essential factor in reducing risk and, consequently, maximising safety, it would seem appropriate to ensure that applicants to work in the UK do have those fluent language skills. For Doctors, working in the UK is governed by registration with the General Medical Council (GMC), who approve applications for those who have passed the tests given by the Professional and Linguistic Assessments Board.

Unfortunately, if an applicant does not speak English, but has lived in another EU country for at least three months, the GMC cannot make the applicant take the test, and must automatically grant them the right to practise as a Doctor. Patient safety, therefore, is compromised, and the only way the non-English speaking Doctor can be removed from the GMC Register is when they have caused harm to a patient. (PATIENTS, if you suspect your doctor does not understand what you say, it may well be the case that they don't understand.)

20: DRUG CALCULATIONS

One of the key safety requirements for registration as a doctor, nurse, or allied health professional (paramedic, anaesthetic technician [ODP]), is the ability to solve any relevant drug calculation problem, regardless of difficulty, without the aid of a calculator, and with one hundred percent accuracy. Without accurate drug calculations, administration of safe drug dosages would not be possible, and patients are MUCH more likely to suffer harm, as a consequence.

To ensure that nurses (etc) have appropriate calculation ability, NHS hospitals make job applicants take drug calculation tests, as part of their interview experience. By all appearances, this is a method of filtering out those professionals who are not properly competent to safely measure or administer drugs. But, once again, this is just propaganda, or "spin", to give the impression that the NHS does ensure that only properly competent staff are employed when, in reality, successful applicants are offered jobs, regardless of whether or not they pass their tests, but because they do not pose any sort of threat to the manager, or because they are of the manager's "favoured" status. This lack of numeracy issue is, in the main, something which the NHS successfully covers up, and any objective studies of the problem are not widely disseminated.

One rare study was conducted, in 2010, by the *Journal of Advanced Nursing*, who found that only 11% of nurses could successfully calculate **basic** drug calculation problems. Subsequently, there have been no changes to the testing or auditing of nurses or anaesthetic technicians, with respect to drug calculation ability, so it is reasonable to assume that there has not been an improvement in standards since the 2010 study.

University Drug Calculation Examinations

An example of how drug calculation ability is more a matter of propaganda and image than assurance of patient safety, is that of the drug calculation exam for anaesthetic technician (Operating Department Practitioner) students. In most instances, the format for this exam is not of the traditional supervised classroom type but, instead, is based on examination via a website, where the student has to register their details, and is given a date by which they are required to successfully pass the online calculation test. Students do not take the test under supervision and scrutiny, but are free to take the test at any place where they have internet access: at home, in the library, on the bus, or on holiday - there are no restrictions, other than the submission date. It does not require much imagination to realise that those individuals, who do not possess the basic numeracy skills necessary to pass the calculation test, are free to use the assistance of friends and family, or any other facility for passing the exams. This, indeed, is what happens. The examinations are fake assessments, which do not test a student's ability, but give the impression that they are part of an overall safety regime. Proof of this situation is very easy to determine through independent testing but, because it would be a vote loser, it is a matter which will never be formally investigated – by a government of any party.

🕮 Registration Requirement

Why then, is drug calculation ability a registration requirement, when most nurses and allied professionals do not possess the skills to perform drug calculation problems? The answer is because it is part of the NHS penchant for positive propaganda.

How can this lack of numeracy problem, amongst professionally registered practitioners, be solved? This is easy to answer; all the government has to do is remove the requirement for drug calculation ability from registration requirements, and make it a separate qualification. In doing so, healthcare delivery will be more honest, transparent, and safe, because only provably competent staff will be involved in calculating drug dosages.

🕮 Job Interview Drug Calculation Testing

☠ The testing regime for clinical job applicants has the same veracity and authenticity as that of the anaesthetic technician student testing system, described above, inasmuch as applicants are pre-warned of **exactly** the type of questions they are to face, usually by means of informing them that the test questions will be taken from a particular web site, such as "www.testandcalc.com".

☠ The mathematical standard for passing calculation tests is very low, and no higher than that for an eleven year old child to pass the "11+" exam, and does not ever include all types of calculation problem which might be encountered; only the simpler types of calculation are posed.

☠ Even with these vary basic tests, most nurses and anaesthetic technicians fail to meet the required standard and, in not a few cases, they do not have the ability to calculate something as fundamental as resolving, for example, 40% of 200.

☠ It would be accurate to say that the vast majority of the subjects taking a meaningful drug calculation test will fail to meet the criteria demanded by their registration, but the people who are recorded as having "passed" are those who the selection panels have already decided they want to employ.

The remaining unsuccessful applicants, who have been informed that they failed their drug calculation tests, will have to accept their failures, because they know that the results are accurate, for them, and they will have no recourse to complain about unfair treatment, lest they attract the attention of their respective registration bodies and, potentially, have their registrations removed because of their drug calculation failings. Successful applicants, on the other hand, will be beholding to the managers or team leaders who have recorded them as having been successful, and their conformity with the NHS cover-up culture will be assured.

🚑 Drug Calculation Propaganda

Essentially, drug calculation tests are twin purpose instruments of career progression, because they provide a manager with justification for not employing or promoting one person, because they failed their drug calculation test, whilst also justifying employing or promoting another employee, because they have been officially recorded as having passed their test, even though they did not score any better than the rejected applicant. Incidentally, with few exceptions, nurses and allied professionals do not perform drug calculations as part of their daily duties, and mathematical ability is not related to nursing ability. Indeed, a nurse who is not so academically gifted is likely to compensate for such a lack by being extra capable and conscientious at standard nursing practices. The reasons why such ability is part of registration requirements, are so that the public will believe that their safety is enhanced, and that more responsibility, when things go wrong, is shifted towards these professionals, and away from management. This drug calculation ability issue is another dirty trick against staff, and does nothing to reduce risk to patients which, itself, means that the Health and Safety at Work Act duty to reduce risk is compromised, so these fake drug calculation competencies increase, rather than reduce, risk to patients.

🚑 Patient Safety Example

When planning for safety, reducing risk is only achieved when mitigating against worst case scenarios which, for drug calculation situations, means a combination of multiple human factors. For example, when a doctor, such as an anaesthetist, has to perform a rare or relatively difficult calculation problem, and has the added difficulties of suffering the adverse effects of stress, fatigue, and distractions, during a busy night shift, and when there is a shortage of staff, the possibility of error is significantly increased, and the error might be as severe as mistaking milligrams for micrograms. To help ensure safety, he/she will be obliged to ask a second qualified person to confirm the validity of the calculated dosage. The anaesthetist will know that drug calculation ability is a professional registration requirement for nurses and anaesthetic technicians and, therefore, will have no hesitation in asking one of these practitioner types to confirm the calculation. The chosen anaesthetic technician (or nurse) may not want to admit a lack of ability in this regard, lest he/she lose their registration, but will recognise that the anaesthetist is highly intelligent, and will assume that their calculation is valid, so will pretend to have confirmed that the calculation is, indeed, correct. If the calculation is incorrect, then safety is compromised, and the patient could suffer severe harm, particularly if they are administered an overdose.

Alternatively, if the technician or nurse was not subject to the registration requirement for drug calculation ability, he/she would be acting properly by declining to validate the anaesthetist's calculation. The anaesthetist would then have to search for someone who does have drug calculation ability, and who will properly and validate the anaesthetists's calculation and, in doing so, would fulfil the requirements of a safe drug administration regime.

The above scenario, which is not an unrealistic one, demonstrates how drug calculation requirements, for nurses and anaesthetic technicians, poses an increased risk to patients.

♣ Dyslexic Healthcare Workers

A lack of numeracy skills is not the only issue which adversely effects safety: readers, who are not familiar with the reality of the NHS, may be surprised to discover that there are nurses and anaesthetic technicians who are dyslexic, even though these jobs require that they are able to read drug labels, blood gas reports, patient care plans, identity bracelets, and blood product labels. Making a mistake, in any of these areas can, and does, result in significant harm to patients but, once more, this dyslexia issue demonstrates the NHS pattern of propaganda, which is aimed at convincing the public of the veracity of clinical qualifications when, in fact, there is no such veracity.

🚑 21: INFECTION CONTROL

Anyone who is interested in some of the reasons why a patient might suffer a hospital acquired infection, or why so many hospital patients suffer harm, including death, from **sepsis**, should read this chapter, which gives an insider's perspective into the practicalities and NHS public relations "spin" concerning hygiene and infection control.

I nfection is one of the most serious hazards posed to patients, particularly in hospital settings, and an estimated 300,000 patients a year acquire a Healthcare Acquired Infection (HCAI), also known as *nosocomial* infection. Infection is not just a problem for health, it also has a financial burden, with an annual cost to taxpayers of over one billion pounds - according to a UK Parliament report: *Raising standards of infection prevention and control in the NHS (House of Commons debate pack, CDP-2018-0116, May 2018).*

🚑 Sepsis

According to the *Septic Alliance*, the main consequence, to patients, of poor hygiene, is the possibility of developing infection, leading to sepsis, which can result in life threatening organ failure, caused by the body's erratic response to infection. Amongst these septic patients, an estimated 48,000 patients (UK Sepsis Trust) die each year, because of their infections, with the main infection types being *Clostridium difficile, Methicillin Resistant Staphylococcus Aureus,* and *Escherichia coli.*

The figure of 48,000 deaths is only one of several official estimates, and it should, in fact, be treated as a minimal value. A more significant estimate is derived from the Standard Hospital Mortality Index (SHMI), which reports that approximately 294,000 patients die, each year, either in hospital, or within 30 days of discharge, with a third of those deaths being caused by sepsis, which brings the patient death figure to nearer 100,000. Clearly the mortality rate of patients, due to sepsis, is not trivial, and that fact is recognised by the World Health Organisation, who report that sepsis is responsible for 1 in 5 deaths worldwide.

⚑ NHS Digital Report on Hospital Death Rates, 2018.

According to this report, the English hospitals with the highest death rates were (worst first)...

Colchester • United Lincolnshire • Royal Wolverhampton • Coventry and Warwickshire • Northern Lincolnshire and Goole • Blackpool • Sandwell and W Birmingham • Wigan and Leigh •

James Paget • Southport and Ormskirk • Wye Valley • Dorset.

The Sepsis Alliance assertion, that one third of UK patient deaths are from sepsis, and poor hygiene, is a principle factor in developing sepsis, means that these hospitals must have poorer hygiene practices than other hospitals. Before considering attending one of these hospitals, therefore, it might be wise to consult the latest mortality figures (online) from the Standard Hospital Mortality Indicator.

🚑 Hand Hygiene

The principle cause of passing infectious agents, or pathogens, to a patient, is transmission by "direct contact", a term which describes both physical contact, and face-to-face interaction. In particular, it is the finger tips which take up pathogens from "reservoirs of infection", and which transfer those pathogens to a patient, or an intermediate settling place which the patient subsequently touches. This is a problem that can be addressed by good general hygiene practices, especially proper hand washing.

The public will be familiar with the frequent press reports concerning sepsis related deaths from healthcare acquired infections, and these reports are usually accompanied by official NHS statements of intent, to rectify the problem, including steps to reduce cross contamination caused by poor hand hygiene.

🚑 Hand Washing

Clinical staff are supposed to be instructed in the ways of proper hand washing and decontamination, as part of basic and ongoing training, with the aim of ensuring that infection control is of an optimum standard, both for the protection of the employee whose skin may be contaminated with pathogens, and for the protection of patients who may become contaminated by that employee, either directly or indirectly.

According to NHS England...

"Good hand hygiene and handwashing techniques, amongst the public and professionals in all sectors (*National Institute of Clinical Excellence: Quality Standard on Infection Control*), will help to reduce the spread of infection, thereby reducing the chances of sepsis developing as a result."

As part of NHS hand washing guidelines, a significant recommendation is that the person washing their hands should not make direct contact with any part of the washing station components, such as soap dispenser, or the tap itself. Instead, the NHS stipulates the use of holding an appropriate hand drying paper towel when dispensing the soap, and when turning the taps on and off. I have never seen any other person complying with this stipulation, and it is not something that is subject to audit, training, or enforcement. Why is this? NHS managers care, primarily, with their own survival and success, and the way they achieve that is to satisfy governement targets. Hand hygiene is not subject to government targets, so it is of no interest to hospital managers.

⏺ BBC Hand Washing Demonstration

As an example of the real world attitude that NHS employers have, regarding proper hand hygiene, the news programme, *BBC Look North*, ran a feature about how Boston Pilgrim Hospital was responding to a national and contemporary problem of patient deaths due to healthcare acquired infections. In this news item, which was meant to be self promoting propaganda for the hospital, the BBC interviewed senior members of staff about the steps they ware taking to deal with this infection problem, and filmed a demonstration of "proper" hand washing technique, by a ward nurse. In this demonstration, the nurse used a sink which was operated with lever arm taps which, because of their high mechanical advantage, require very little force to turn the water flows on or off. The purpose of such a system is to minimise the effort required by users, and allow them to avoid using their fingers to adjust the water flow and, instead, use their elbows, which offer a much smaller risk of cross contamination than fingers do.

Upon approaching the sink, the nurse pulled the lever arms, with her bare fingers, to turn on the hot and cold water supplies. After washing her hands, the nurse turned off the water flows, once again using her bare and newly cleaned fingers. She then dried her hands with paper towels. There are a number of points to note about the stages of this televised hand washing demonstration:

1) By turning the taps on, with her bare fingers, any pathogens on her fingers were transferred to the taps.

2) If her hand washing technique was effective, the pathogens on her fingers would have been removed, and flushed safely away.

3) By using her fingers, again, to turn the taps off, the nurse recontaminated her fingers with the same pathogens which were present before she washed her hands.

4) In addition to recontaminating her hands with her original pathogens, the nurse would have added to that contamination with pathogens already on the taps, and which were previously deposited by other members of staff.

5) By complying with the hospital hand washing method, the nurse's hands were <u>more</u> contaminated after the hand washing process, than they were beforehand.

The above account is an example of propaganda gone wrong – the hospital wanted to reassure the public that clinical staff protected patients with their rigorous hand washing routine but, instead, they inadvertently gave a very public demonstration of a washing routine which actually INCREASED risk to patients.

Note: Readers should not consider this hospital's infection control protocol as an isolated example of why healthcare acquired infections occur, but should treat it for what it really is, which is an example of "professionalism", generally, in the NHS, where the attitude is, if something does not involve a government target, then do not give it much thought or analysis.

🔌 National Institute for Health and Care Excellence

In their *Quality Standards and Indicators* briefing paper, the National Institute for Health and Care Excellence (NICE) recommends regular hand hygiene audits, over twenty-four hour periods, using multiple sources of data, which means comprehensive investigations into hygiene practices. NICE also recommends that the results of hand hygiene audits be made available to employees, as a source of feedback about their compliance levels. In reality, such audits are so rarely conducted, that most clinical staff would probably say that hand hygiene audits "never happen".

At one exceptional and covertly executed hand hygiene audit, of a Hampshire hospital, investigators reported (to NICE) hygiene compliance in clinical hand-touch events at no better than 25%. This figure matched that of an investigation at the same hospital, two years previously, which suggests that no changes were made to improve hand hygiene compliance since that earlier audit. This is unsurprising, because hospital directors and managers are uncomfortable with change; they do not want to commission fixes to problems, such as poor hand hygiene, because that would mean admitting that problems exist – they prefer not to see or hear about problems – a characteristic of the cover-up culture of the NHS.

Incidentally, whilst working in operating theatres, I have never seen anyone – Doctor, Nurse, HCA, or Anaesthetic Technician – wash their hands "between" patients, unless there was extraordinary reason to, such as when their hands were obviously contaminated with blood.

Infection Issues

♨ Coughing and Sneezing

From an early age, children are taught that "coughs and sneezes spread diseases", yet a majority of NHS clinical staff take no notice of this adage. They will sneeze and cough over food and people, use their bare hands to wipe away expectorated substances from their mouths and noses, and will not subsequently wash their hands. I once witnessed a sneeze by a person standing at one end of a staff room dinner table, when the light, behind me, highlighted the particles in the air, including the mucous sneezed out by this person, some of which sprayed the diners, and the rest travelled to the notice board on the facing wall, which was over five yards (five metres) away. When I pointed this out, to the sneezer, his reply was "Philippino snot is okay, it is like honey. Ha! Ha!".

All this disregard for hygiene is despite NHS England producing television public information messages, and easily accessible posters, declaring that "Germs can live for several hours on tissues, so dispose of them as soon as possible", and "Hands can transfer germs to every surface you touch, so clean them straight away". To emphasise this message, both to clinical staff and the general public, these sentiments are encapsulated with the mantra of:

Catch it. Bin it. Kill it.

Still, the message goes unheard. Either staff do not understand the issue, or they just do not care.

☺ Finger Licking

Another disgusting and dangerous habit, possessed by some staff, at all levels, from the most junior health care assistant, to the most senior Consultant, is that of using finger licked mucus as lubrication, when leafing through sheaves of papers. By itself, transferring one's spit to the fingers, which then touch other objects, or people, should be treated as a serious breach of infection control protocols, but the problem goes even further, and some readers might find it difficult to believe what I describe next:

When some surgeons examine a patient, they will poke and prod the patient, with their bare hands, and feel around the surgical target area. They do not follow the general rule to wash their hands

immediately before and **immediately** after patient contact, or to don gloves. A particularly unpleasant example of this commonly practiced phenomenon is that of a surgeon who examined a day case patient, who was to be treated for a peri-anal cyst. After probing around this patient's anal and inner buttock areas, and poking and squeezing the cyst, with his bare fingers, the surgeon moved to a work station to leaf through the patient's clinical notes, licking his fingers before every page turn. After reading through the notes, the surgeon modified the patient's clinical computer records and, by so doing, contaminated the computer keyboard with whatever pathogens he picked up from the patient's anal area. The "nurse in charge" of the operating theatre cleaned everything she could see that the surgeon touched, but she did not raise this as an issue because, as she said, "I have a mortgage to pay".

♨ Staff Screening

NHS employment candidates are screened for, and vaccinated against, various contagious conditions, such as Hepatitis B/C, Measles, and Rubella; once employed, these screened employees are deemed "safe" to work in clinical environments. Such screening, however, is limited, and very much "one off" events, and there are no protocols for ongoing screening of staff for infectious conditions. This shows a serious lack of regard for safety, because properly screened staff can subsequently become contaminated with other agents, either from patients or from the external environment, and those staff, in turn, can contaminate patients.

A prime example of this scenario occurs with staff who take their holidays in countries where contagion of dangerous and endemic diseases is a real threat. This situation occurred in 2016, during a large Ebola outbreak in parts of West Africa, mostly in Sierra Leone and Liberia: A "scrub" nurse, from a large London hospital, took her annual three week holiday in her home country, Sierra Leone, during this Ebola outbreak. Upon return to the UK, there was no requirement for her to be screened for Ebola or, indeed, any other contagious agent, before resuming her duties as a surgical scrub nurse. Fortunately, she did not pick up a disease condition in Africa, but the fact that this nurse was not infected did not mean that she did not pose a risk. The Health and Safety at Work Act is clear on this point (Precautionary Principle); it is the potential risk that has to be recognised and mitigated against. Hoping that a contagion event does not occur does not comply with British safety legislation, neither does it satisfy the principles of common sense. This non precautionary approach is a very British attitude to safety: do not accept that a hazard exists, until someone is harmed, before accepting that the hazard does, indeed, exist.

To put this staff health screening situation in a contemporary context, compare it with the practice of cladding buildings with inflammable materials, prior to the London Grenfell Tower fire, in 2017. Before the fire, national and local government bodies decreed those cladding materials to be safe, because nobody had died as a result of their use. After the fire, that particular cladding material was ruled to be dangerous, because people did die as a consequence of its use, and it was quickly banned for use as building cladding.

Waiting for a dangerous event to occur, such as with the Grenfell fire, or the nurse visiting a country rife with contagion, before using it as evidence of a real hazard, is not true safety, which should be "proactive", but fake safety, because it is "reactive", and because it occurs after someone comes to harm.

⚅ Hospital Cleaning

Systematic cleaning is a key component of anti-contamination protocols. In a hospital, cleaning and waste disposal are so central to effective healthcare that, should these systems fail, safe healthcare delivery would not be possible, and the hospital would have to close down. Clearly, cleaning services should be considered to have the highest priority, if safe healthcare services are to be delivered, and complied with by the most junior porter, to the most senior board members and Chief Executive. In practice, cleaning is just something which happens - there is no great management interest in the subject, other than producing related documents and guidelines to give the impression that it is something which is taken seriously.

In some NHS hospitals, cleaning and hygiene are executed at a less than minimalist level, and nobody with power of office wants to make any serious attempt at correcting this situation, because it makes "bad news" for the hospital, and its Chief Executive.

⚅ NHS National Specifications for Cleanliness, 2004.

These specifications, produced by the NHS *National Patient Safety Agency*, are meant to ensure that cleaning services are adequately resourced, and set and measure performance outcomes for both in-house and contract cleaning services, with the object of lowering the rates of healthcare acquired infections.

As part of the specification, hospital areas are classed according to functional risk, and the higher risk areas require higher emphasis for cleaning and infection control. Those areas which are classed as **functionally high risk** include: Operating Theatres, Intensive Care Units, Accident and Emergency (A&E) departments, and other departments where invasive procedures are performed or where, immuno-compromised patients receive care. Additionally, the functionally high risk category is applied to areas adjoining the above functionally high risk areas, including staff lounges, toilets, and offices. In line with the way things work in the NHS, cleaners are hardly ever seen cleaning these staff areas, especially in the highest risk area, which is operating theatre departments, even though providing safe and clean staff facilities is a mandatory requirement of the *Welfare at Work Regulations*. In NHS hospitals, clean staff changing rooms do not exist, and a staff eating area can be as disgusting as a squat for drug addicts.

✎ Specific Targets of Cleaning

The NHS *Cleanliness Specifications* provides examples of high risk objects which should be subject to regular cleaning, including:

> Drip stands, pulse oximeters, infusion pumps, electrical equipment and sockets and switches, walls, ceilings, chairs, tables, doors, door handles and push plates, internal glazing, hygiene dispensers, and ventilation grilles.

It would be accurate to say that there is virtually never any cleaning of these items, and no published local policies, guidelines, or audits for such cleaning. The *NHS National Specifications for Cleanliness,* appears to be more "spin" than substance, and is part of the concealment tradition of the NHS.

📖 Outsourced Cleaning

In most NHS hospitals, the cleaning function is outsourced to private companies who, because they are profit making enterprises, are driven by making money, which is their "raison d'être", and not by providing the best possible cleaning service.

Before winning a hospital cleaning contract, a cleaning company has to compete with other cleaning companies, and must guarantee delivery of services for a fixed price and, to win the contract, the company has to bid a lower price than its competitors. For example, at one hospital, the winning company won the hospital's cleaning contract because the price in their bid was approximately eight million pounds lower than the next lowest bidder. With such a low price, which is fixed, the only way the company can maximise their profit, is by minimising costs, and the main way that is accomplished is by minimising the payroll. This, is, indeed, what they do.

Cleaning company employees are poorly paid (as most U.K. workers are), and the number of employees is kept at the minimum possible, rather than being decided by what number would deliver the best possible cleaning service. To ensure a compliant workforce (there are lots of things to be kept hidden), cleaning company employees are either illegal immigrants, or do not possess the necessary English language skills to take up any other lines of work. These people will never blow the whistle on matters which are of public concern, because they are trapped in their situations, and this makes them compliant with the extended cover-up culture of the NHS. Being trapped in their jobs, especially for the illegal immigrants, is also why these employees have to comply with demands to do unpaid overtime, which is a way for the company to minimise the number of people they employ and hence, reduce costs and increase profits.

Incidentally, the above-mentioned job entrapment is one of the definitions of **modern slavery**. (As an aside, most private hospitals do not outsource the cleaning function - they employ cleaners directly - and their hygiene standards are significantly superior to NHS hospitals, both in patient and staff areas.)

If the NHS is to pontificate on standards for hygiene, cleaning, and infection control practices, then it must also ensure that there is compliance with those standards, and <u>independent</u> auditing of such, which it does not do, and which is why sepsis continues to be a significant threat to patient safety.

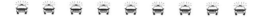

22: EXAMPLE INFECTION RISK

A memorable example of why the NHS has such a poor record of protecting patients from infection, is that of something that I discovered when doing a locum shift at the Royal Free hospital, Belsize Park, London. This concerned one of the anaesthetic nurses, who was well known as being someone who was unfriendly and uncooperative, and who hated his job, because he had to follow instructions from women and non-muslims, something that he found deeply offensive.

With respect to infection control, he, the anaesthetic nurse, took a lot of short-cuts, such as not washing his hands after visiting the toilet, or before and after patient contact. He would also sign the anaesthetic room daily cleaning journal, without doing anything other than cleaning visible signs of contamination, such as blood. The issue, addressed here, concerns that of failure to decontaminate bronchoscopes.

<u>Note</u>: A bronchoscope is a flexible cable, with a remotely manoeuvrable camera at the end. The scope is passed through the patient's mouth and windpipe, into a lung, so that the surgeon and or anaesthetist can locate problems such as tumours. After being used, the scope will be covered in blood and secretions, and must undergo manufacturer instructions for cleaning and sterilisation, using

specially provided agents and processes.

This particular anaesthetic nurse, through laziness and nastiness, would not bother to follow the proper bronchoscope decontamination protocol. Instead, he would just wipe away the visible blood and mucous secretions, using a paper towel from an above sink dispenser. He did not care about the consequences to a patient of having traces of someone else's blood and secretions deposited into their respiratory tract. (Behavioural Psychologists might have a label for the nurse's behaviour, but the average person might reasonably regard him as being psychopathic.)

Many of the staff, who witnessed his actions, would discuss the nurse's behaviour amongst themselves, but were too scared to report him, because he was large and intimidating, and they knew that he would be told who the "snitch" was. The theatre department manager, typically, did not want to hear about this issue, because NHS managers function with a "hear no evil, see no evil" attitude, but it was commonly known that she knew what was going on.

Eventually, one of the anaesthetists noticed that a bronchoscope, packed and labelled as clean, had traces of dried blood on it, so he informed the manager of the fact. The manager could no longer avoid addressing this important matter of infection control because, otherwise, the gossip network would work against her. To everyone's disgust, however, the manager chose not to speak with the nurse, but decided, instead, to protect herself from his inevitable accusations, against her, of being anti-muslim, or discriminating against him for being the only Jordanian in the department, so she printed out laminated bronchoscope cleaning instructions, and posted one sheet in each anaesthetic room, and left it at that. Subsequently, most of the

other anaesthetic nurses and operating department practitioners assumed the habit of cleaning the bronchoscopes both before and after use.

📖　📖　📖　📖　📖

For the reader, who does not have experience of working in the NHS, the above account may seem unbelievable or, at least, a very rare situation. Most clinical NHS staff, however, particularly the experienced ones, will attest to similar and even worse accounts of dangerous and disgusting behaviours that pose a threat to patient safety. Of those people – doctors, nurses, paramedics, anaesthetic technicians - the ones who speak out about those instances, and become whistleblowers, are the ones who do not get the promotion and other career opportunities that they deserve. Indeed they suffer retribution that permanently labels them as trouble makers, and scars them, mentally, to the extent that, eventually, their resistance to health problems is diminished and, in some cases, the induced depression pushes to them to commit, or at least to consider, suicide. The NHS is a brutal organisation.

23: BULLYING & HARASSMENT

When an NHS employee experiences unwanted treatment by a bullying colleague, or a manager, it might be for any of several reasons which, commonly, are:

❶ Personal animosity

❷ Rejecting a sexual predator

❸ They pose a professional threat to the bully

❹ They pose a threat to the manager's position

① Personal animosity can be due to discrimination, or because the bully is jealous of their victim, perhaps because the victim has greater potential for career progress. If the issue is discrimination, then this is more of an issue of harassment than bullying.

② In the NHS, it is common for staff to gain career progression through voluntarily establishing sexual relationships with senior staff who have the power to reward them with job protection, specialist training, promotion, and so on. Typically, the senior person will be male, and the responsive junior will be an unmarried female, with little in the way of ability, intelligence, or professional attitude - they take the easy and quick route to career progression. In some cases, the target of the predatory behaviour will refuse to become involved with this type of behaviour and, as a result, will suffer career sabotage, using such techniques as gaslighting and social isolation. These victims of predation will seek help from senior females, their union, or Freedom To Speak Up Guardian, but will NEVER be helped by any of these or other officials who are meant to protect them from bullying and sexual harassment. Indeed, they are much more likely to join in with the bullying, in the hope that they can close down (cover up) the matter.

③ Being a threat occurs when the bully feels that their victim may discover some inadequacy in the bully's qualifications, or unsuitability for their role. This is a common problem, because many NHS employees do not have the competence to comply with their registration requirements, Another potential threat, to the bully, occurs when the bully has some personal issue to hide, such as drug abuse, and they believe that their victim might be astute enough to discover their secret, so they mitigate the problem by distracting and intimidating them with bullying.

④ If a nurse (etc) is not the type of person who a manager can force into complying with the department's cover-up culture and, because of that, poses a threat to the manager's position, they are most likely to fall victim of bullying, either by being denied career advancement and support, or by using the victim's colleagues as proxy bullies. There are plenty of obsequious employees in the NHS, who will plot against their colleagues, and become willing bullies, in order to gain favour with a manager, and that is how many undeserving people achieve promotion, by doing whatever is necessary to remove threats to the manager. I have first hand experience of these frauds and drug users, and they were all promoted to senior positions because their "secrets" made them loyal to the NHS cover-up culture, because they benefitted from that same culture.

* * *

Any negative treatment against an employee can be classed as either harassment or bullying; defined as follows:

⚭ Definitions

♟ Harassment

The *NHS Employers* organisation defines harassment as:

> "Unwanted conduct affecting the dignity of anyone in the workplace."

The unwanted conduct may be, for example, sexual harassment, or because of a *protected title* (age etc). It should be noted that the victim is not required to provide independently verifiable proof of the harassment they are subject to – it is their perception of how they are harassed which is of prime concern.

♟ Bullying

> **NHS Employers definition of bullying:**
> "Offensive, intimidating, malicious or insulting behaviour, an abuse or misuse of power through means intended to undermine, humiliate, denigrate or injure the recipient."

Examples of bullying behaviour include: insults, provocations, social exclusion, unequal or unfair treatment, spreading malicious rumours about the victim, and career sabotage.

♣ The Lord Francis Report, 2013

In his report into the high number of patient deaths at the Mid Staffordshire Trust hospitals, Lord Francis revealed that NHS staff, who blow the whistle on poor practices, are routinely ignored, bullied, and intimidated for raising concerns. Lord Francis also postulated that the NHS uses a climate of fear and intimidation for staff who want to speak out about poor safety and patient care and, during his enquiry, Lord Francis also discovered "shocking" accounts of how whistleblowers are treated. Since publication of the Francis Report, the Department of Health have announced their determination to end the cover-up culture of the NHS, but these announcements are part of the suite of knee-jerk propaganda statements that are normal for the government - the cover-up culture of the NHS is as entrenched now as it always has been.

♨ Victims of Bullying and Harassment

When an employee is subject to harassment or bullying, it can be very difficult for them to deal with the problem or, indeed, to understand how or why they are being treated in such a way. If, for example, the employee senses that some staff appear to be hostile toward them, it could be because someone has been poisoning the minds of their colleagues by spreading malicious gossip against them, and the victim may never discover or even suspect that this is the cause of their discomfort. Alternatively, an individual might be very forward and direct in their negative conduct against their victim but, without independent and reliable witnesses to the harassing or bullying behaviour, they (the victim) might not see any avenue which might lead to halting that unwanted behaviour.

An understanding of how harassment and bullying are defined and realised can make it possible for the victim to better understand who the beneficiaries of the harassment and bullying are, and what their motivations could be. Identifying a bully is the first task, and is generally not difficult; aggressive bullies are often physically larger than their victims, have poor social skills (no manners), weak communication ability (small vocabulary), and have lower intelligence than their colleagues. These people also tend to put much effort into ingratiating themselves with senior staff, because they are not adequately competent for their roles, and being "friends" with managers, and doing favours for them (as agent provocateurs) is the only way they can make career progress.

Armed with such knowledge, the victim of bullying and harassment can be much better equipped to make official (written) protestations against who is responsible for their suffering, and the motivations they might have. By doing so, the victim is unlikely to be properly or fairly protected by management, especially as raising the issue of any type of bullying is something that managers and personnel department clerks will want suppressed, but speaking out does put into view whatever it is that is being covered-up, or whomever is motivated to bully or harass the victim. Essentially, when the bullying victim knows who is the cause of their unfair treatment, and the reasons and motivations for that treatment, and they are prepared to speak out about the issue, they will weaken the resolve of their persecutors because, invariably, the perpetrators will have something about them that they want to remain concealed, such as their dubious qualifications and professional suitability for their posts, what issues they have previously covered up, or their personal habits - particularly if they are drug users. These people do not want to attract attention to themselves.

The reason why I specifically mention drug use is because it is a very widespread problem amongst NHS employees, and those drug users are never low key individuals; they are always looking for strategic alliances with senior staff who might, one day, be able to protect them from investigations into their personal habits.

Note: A useful clue that someone might have something to hide - drugs, qualifications etc - is that they will ingratiate themselves with specific groups or managers, by bullying or harassing individuals on behalf of those groups or managers. In effect, they become willing and unprompted proxy bullies for their potential protectors. This phenomenon may not be unique to the NHS, but it is certainly ubiquitous within the NHS.

Bullying Dirty Tricks

When an NHS employee is subject to bullying or harassment, and has the fortitude to make official protestations about the abuse they suffer, they can expect to become subject to less direct and more impersonal "dirty tricks" which will make their employment more uncomfortable and less secure. Three dirty tricks of note, because they are not so easy to prove, but are commonly used, are:

♣ Sabotage

In clinical areas, there is always equipment to check, and other patient related preparations to make. When an employee, such as a nurse or anaesthetic technician wants to indirectly bully a colleague (the victim), they can, and do, cause trouble for them by sabotaging their work areas, such as modifying or removing equipment which their victim has previously prepared and checked. The aim of such sabotage is to cause the victim to be disciplined for failing to properly prepare their work area. The fact that such sabotage can increase risk to patients is of no concern to the saboteur, especially when the saboteur is a drug user, because these people are either desperate, or not in complete control of their actions.

Some examples of sabotage, in operating theatres, include:

● Removing endotracheal tube introducers, which are absolutely essential for patient safety, from an anaesthetic technician's or anaesthetic nurse's work area.

● Replacing laryngoscope batteries with "dead" batteries.

● Cutting very small slits in a breathing circuit, after it has been tested for leaks. Consequently, the breathing circuit will not function safely, and that poses a risk to a patient.

● Removing or damaging essential patient monitoring components. This causes delays in patient care, whilst new monitoring components are hunted down.

● Moving drug ampoules of one type to a box of another type, where the labels are similar in design and colour, in the hope that the victim will issue the wrong drug to the anaesthetist.

In each of the above cases, patient safety is compromised, but the saboteur does not care about that, because their objective is to ensure that their victim is accused of being unsafe and unprofessional.

♣ Talk to the Bully

Hospitals produce anti-harassment and anti-bullying policies, which include the *speak to the bully first* policy that a victim of bullying or harassment speak to their attacker, before considering making an official complaint against them. The given reason for this policy is to try to resolve any differences, so that official disciplinary Hearings can be avoided, and everyone can continue their work in a happy and positive manner.

The real and unofficial reason for this policy is to portray the hospital as following the principles of reasonableness, compassion, and generosity between employees. In reality, the consequence of "speaking to the bully first" is that the bully will, immediately after being spoken to, make an official complaint against their victim, and accuse them of being aggressive and threatening, thereby making the bully seem like the victim. Thus, the bullying campaign against the real bullying victim accelerates.

♣ Mediation

Another management trick, to suppress a bullying victim's attempts to put a halt to their bullying, is to discourage them from formally reporting the bully and, instead, encourage them to attend a meeting with the bully, and a mediator, to resolve the problem. The official aim of the meeting is to allow an informal resolution to the problem between the bully and their victim.

When the bullied victim attends a mediation meeting, they might assume that the mediation process is a legitimate and fair method of putting a stop to the stopping. If that were not the case, they would not agree to mediation, and would insist on moving straight to the formal complaints protocol. What the victim will not realise, at least at the time of the mediation, is that the mediator, who is supposed to be impartial, is there to protect the professional image of the bullying victim's manager, and that is achieved by deterring the victim from proceeding on to the formal complaints process against the bully.

The real aims of mediation are any combination of:

❂ Protect the leadership reputation of the victim's manager, by "converting" a complaint of bullying into an informal discussion.

❂ Allow the bully to protest their innocence.

❂ "Gaslight" the victim into thinking that they are being overly sensitive, unreasonable, or they have misinterpreted the other person's behaviour.

❂ Enable counter claims of unreasonable behaviour against the victim, should they not allow the mediation meeting to settle the bullying claim.

❂ Make the claim, real or otherwise, that the victim is being unduly emotional, and is incapable of being rational and reasonable. This method of accusing the victim of failing to be subjective and calm is known as *tone policing*, or *tone fallacy*, and is a way of deflecting from the victim's problem, and towards the victim's character – it is a technique of maskirovka, as described in Appendix 2.

Mediation is, itself, a surreptitious method of bullying, and a controlling process that helps to enforce the cover-up culture that management depend on for their own career survival and success.

♠ Dead Cat Strategy

If an employee makes a complaint against a harassing colleague, manager or team leader, the departmental manager, with advice from personnel department clerks, might deflect attention from the particular issue by using the "dead cat strategy", which means introducing another subject which overwhelms the original issue, and makes it difficult for the injured person to continue with their original complaint. A simple example would be that of introducing the claim that the victim was frightened that the other person (the bully) was about to report the victim for incompetence, and making the accusation of bullying was a way of deterring such complaints of lack of competence from being made.

Another example of a dead cat strategy, which is commonly and effectively used against male employees who makes complaints against female colleagues, is to close down the complaint by suggesting that the male employee is a mysogynist. Male employees have no defence against such an accusation and, unless they terminate their original complaint against the female harasser, they will be the ones who experience disciplinary action.

♠ Staff Appraisal

To satisfy the imperative of maintaining the cover-up culture, NHS employers use the surreptitious process of annual staff appraisal, where a staff member is subject to professional scrutiny from their team leader or manager. Officially, appraisal is meant to identify strengths and weaknesses of employees, and helps guide individual professional progress, with such things as further training, or support with certain tasks. If the appraisal is a negative one, then the staff member's career prospects will be curtailed, and chances of promotion or further training will be stymied. As a consequence, the employee will always feel subdued and constrained, with respect to making complaints about the manager who gives their appraisals and, if the manager is involved in fraud, drug use, favouritism, discrimination, or is incompetent, reporting the manager will result in a poor appraisal for the employee making the complaint.

The whole appraisal scheme is really just another aspect of maskirovka, where the real purpose – suppressing whistleblowers – is masked by the appraisal methodology of Personnel Management, which serves to make the organisation appear to be proactive in staff development, but is really only a "front" for intimidation and control.

♣ DARVO

DARVO is an acronym for **D**eny, **A**ttack, **R**everse, **V**ictim, **O**ffender, and was created by psychology Professor Jennifer Freyd (1997) of the University of Oregon. DARVO describes the reaction of a perpetrator of, for example, bullying, in order to avoid being held accountable for their actions.

♟ Deny: The bully denies their bullying behaviour.

♟ Attack: The bully counters accusations from their victim by making false counter accusations against them, **Attacking** their credibility, and putting them on the defensive.

♟ Reverse: The bully attempts to reverse the roles of Victim and Offender, by making them seem like the falsely accused victim, and the real victim seem like the real bully/attacker.

In the NHS, when a bullying victim reports their bully to a manager, the bully will **always** use the DARVO tactic which, typically, will be accusations of sexism, racism, or aggression. In some cases, a bully may accuse the person they bullied of being the bully, in an attempt at role reversal.

The DARVO defence is used very successfully against victims of bullying, because managers do not want to have to deal with discrimination or similar matters, in case they lead to adverse publicity against the hospital, and the consequent damage to its reputation. In many cases, the manager takes the side of the bully, because the bully (proxy bully) is loyal to the manager, and the manager's cover-up practices, whereas the victim of bullying might be seen as a threat to the manager.

♟ Staff Surveys

The NHS cover-up culture is made possible by oppressing staff, who might be tempted to raise concerns that might threaten the image of the hospital, and suppressing those employees who have already taken the option of whistleblowing, anonymously. To help identify staff who are at risk of whistleblowing, or have already done so, hospitals use the ruse of pretending to want to listen to their concerns, by commissioning staff surveys.

The surveys are advertised as being impartial, independent, confidential, and anonymous, so that staff feel assured that they cannot be punished or harassed for voicing their concerns. To ensure anonymity, the online survey forms are sent to the email address of each member of staff, along with a unique survey code, which is used in correspondence, instead of using the staff member's name. To generate a unique survey code, and send the questionnaire to a member of staff, the survey system has to be provided with the email addresses of each member of staff, which means the survey team knows who returned a particular questionnaire. Contrary to the claims of anonymity, the identity of the person who submitted a particular questionnaire is known by the hospital (personnel department). Whether this type surreptitious scheme can be classed as fraud is debatable, but it is certainly immoral, and runs contrary to the basic human right of freedom of opinion and expression.

♣ Schwartz Rounds

One other method of discovering who potential whistleblowers are, is the use of pseudo therapy and "sharing" sessions, known as *Schwartz Rounds*, where staff are absorbed into "reflective practice" groups to share their concerns with their peers and *Freedom To Speak Up* (FTSU) Guardians. These are happy clappy style self-congratulatory meetings that aim to make staff feel that their concerns are valued and will be actioned. The truth is that Schwarts Rounds allow managers and FTSU Guardians to learn what issues are in need of the NHS cover-up treatment, who the potential whistleblowers are, and what threats those potential whistleblowers pose to their employers, and to the NHS cover-up culture.

🔊 Staff on Medication

The endemic bullying and cover-up culture of the NHS causes a large proportion of staff, particularly nurses, to suffer long lasting and debilitating stress. Stress is a factor in degraded mental health, but the NHS does not do anything to help employees who are victims of stress, and management do not show any concern with how to address the causes of the stress, even when an employee expressly articulates the cause which, typically, will be unfair or unequal treatment, or being forced into complying with covering up patient safety or related issues.

To manage their stress, many employees will resort to medication, which may or may not be prescribed. In terms of safety, forcing employees to continue performing their clinical duties, whilst suffering stress, and being under the influence of medication, does not meet the legal obligation to reduce risk. The NHS, therefore, contributes to its poor safety culture through neglect of its greatest asset, which is its staff.

🔊 Staff Suicides

An average of 101 NHS staff commit suicide each year, which is an accurate reflection of how the NHS treats its staff, particularly nurses and doctors. According to government research, nurses are 23%

more likely to commit suicide than other members of society, with the prime causal factor being stress, resulting from bullying.

Examples of nurses who have been so overwhelmed by stress that they resorted to suicide include:

Rhian Collins

https://nurse.org/articles/nurse-commits-suicide-bullying/

Leona Goddard

https://www.thesun.co.uk/news/10387836/nhs-nurse-suicide-hospital-stress/

Lucy de Oliveira

https://www.mirror.co.uk/news/uk-news/more-300-overworked-nhs-nurses-14822382

Laura Hyde

https://www.plymouthherald.co.uk/news/plymouth-news/plymouth-woman-one-305-nhs-2813060

Doctors can be victims of bullying and scapegoating as much as nurses can be, in many cases, even more so. When the NHS attacks someone, they do not discriminate – they treat everyone with equal hostility. Suicide, amongst doctors, is such a common problem that the NHS has a website to offer advice to those who need it:

https://php.nhs.uk/resources/suicide-in-doctors/

The general public may find it difficult to understand why so many NHS workers resort to suicide, but the bullying, discrimination, and scapegoating, by hospital directors, managers, and other NHS officials must be experienced to be understood and appreciated. As President Roosevelt said: "You have to be in the gutter, if you want to see the shit floating by".

♣ British Members of Parliament

It is worth making the observation that the suicide rate amongst MPs is so low that it can be considered a "never event". Clearly, stress levels for NHS staff is higher than it is for MPs, and that is one reason why politicians have no genuine interest in this matter – suicide is not a problem that affects them, so they do not care.

🐞 Bullying Anomalies

When considering the issue of bullying, it is also necessary to preempt making conclusions about specific instances without firstly considering the following tangential aspects of bullying:

♣ Unnatural Bully

Some people, including some managers, behave in a way that is neither friendly or unfriendly, they might prefer their own company to others, and make little effort to being diplomatic or supportive of their colleagues. These might be natural character traits for the individual, probably shaped by their upbringing, over which they would have had no control. Alternatively, the character traits may have been learnt through, for example, personal trauma, to themselves or their family, and they may have been scarred by their experiences, with the result that they can be wrongly viewed as having the characteristics of a bully. Once they have been labelled as such, it is common practice, in the NHS, for "everyone" to consider their interaction with the perceived bully as being one where they are being treated in a bullying manner. Thus, the traumatised worker becomes, in the eyes of their colleagues, a genuine bully. This is the herd mentality that permeates the NHS.

♣ Malicious Accusations

There are many people, in the NHS, who do not understand the proper relationship manager:worker relationship. Some people will refuse to follow instructions, however reasonable they are, and will make every effort to disregard rules and regulations, and will not take part in the normally accepted definition of teamwork. Predictably, these people will also refuse to accept criticisms of how they perform their duties, and will have no interest in their contribution to service delivery. To protect themselves against any sort of official sanction, these hostile workers may make accusations of bullying against their manager, and may exaggerate their imagined suffering with false claims of personal animosity or discrimination. The end result can be that the manager has to treat the accuser with kid gloves, other team members have to assume the work duties of the accusing employee, and the effectiveness and morale of the team are undermined by that one person.

♣ Defensive Accusations

Another type of false accusation of bullying that NHS staff can be confronted with, is that from the incompetent or fraudulently registered or falsely qualified individual, who uses accusations of being bullied as a way of donning the persona of someone who is victimised (the DARVO technique). By doing so, they will be able to counter accusations of their lack of ability to do their job properly, so that, eventually, the easiest thing that management can do is to ensure that they are only given the most simple and least responsible tasks to perform.

> In the NHS, bullying is widespread, and permeates all levels of all disciplines, but not all claims of bullying are genuine.

🚍 NHS Highland

The Sturrock Review (2018) into bullying and whistleblowing at the NHS Highland Trust provides a number of descriptions of how top-down bullying is realised in the NHS, and gives personal accounts from senior clinicians of the intimidatory environment in which they had to function. Three sections of the review, that comprehensively illustrate the culture at NHS Highland, including clear assignment of the culpability for the bullying culture being given to the Chief Executive and Directors, follow:

♟ Quote from a Senior Clinician about Board Meetings

"The methods of ambush, intimidation, isolation and undermining reflect the themes raised by those who requested an investigation into bullying at NHS Highland. It demonstrated a Board that is not listening to the concerns of its staff, is driven by its own agenda, and believing itself to be above the law."

♣ Bullying Victim's Account of Indirect Bullying Tactics

"There is persistent inappropriate use of suspension and capability assessments, breaches of confidentiality, and loss of impartiality. This leads to polarisation, tension, stress, unhappiness, sickness and other detriment in individual departments."

♣ Gaslighting

"Gaslighting" is the term to describe the process of persistently and insidiously making a victim lose their sense of reality, question their own beliefs, or convince them that they have a persecution complex, or unreliable memory, in order to psychologically weaken them.

Gaslighting is a commonly used technique that officials use against staff who pose a threat to management, particularly for raising issues that managers prefer to remain hidden. For example, investigations into bullying at NHS Highland emphasise how clinical staff, who have raised issues of concern, have been responded to, by management, with gaslighting techniques of "persistent denial, misdirection, contradiction, and lies, in attempts to destabilise the victims and delegitimize their beliefs".

For patients, who are victims of medical negligence, gaslighting methods can include denial of conversations, replacing original medical notes with forgeries that disprove the negligence, and accusations of being too emotional to understand their cases.

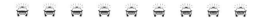

🚑 24: FREEDOM TO SPEAK UP

The failure of the Public Interest Disclosure Act (PIDA) to protect NHS employees from raising concerns was addressed by the Lord Francis Report into the Mid Staffordshire Foundation Trust scandal of 2013. The Report revealed that, essentially, the PIDA is no more than a tool of propaganda, which is meant to convince the public that NHS staff have no barriers to raising issues of public interest when, in fact, those employees who do "blow the whistle" are targeted for retribution to the same degree that they were before the PIDA was introduced.

As with any other issue that undermines the public's trust in the government's ability to effectively manage the NHS, the government had to assure voters of their commitment to the NHS, and so acted on Lord Francis's subsequent recommendation to introduce the concept of having *Freedom To Speak Up Guardians*, so that NHS employees would have a formal and officially accepted route through which they could report their concerns. Consequently, the Department of Health have instructed all hospitals to assign *Freedom To Speak Up Guardians*, with the aim:

"To improve safety and make the health service a better place to work, we need leadership and a culture that places less emphasis on blame when things go wrong, and more importance on transparency and learning from mistakes in the NHS. We require organisations to demonstrate that speaking up is celebrated, and used to address errors or failings, and make improvements that turn 'good' practice into 'great'." **NHS Education England, 2014.**

Hospitals do not have the option of not introducing *Freedom To Speak Up Guardians*, so they embrace their introduction, publically, via their websites, press releases, and public relations pamphlets. One particular hospital has a web page which states:

"It's important to emphasise that staff will not be penalised for raising concerns; they will not lose their job or suffer any form of reprisal. We will not tolerate the harassment or bullying of anyone raising a concern. Nor, will we tolerate any attempt to bully anyone into not raising a concern. Any such behaviour is a breach of our values and, if upheld following investigation, could result in disciplinary action against the perpetrators."

The message that the above statement is trying to convey is that the hospital complies with the law, as required by the Public Interest Disclosure Act. In reality, the message is just one element of the overall rhetorical sales talk that every NHS hospital shares, but it is without substance.

The efficacy of *Freedom To Speak Up Guardians* can be measured by its effectiveness in protecting employees who have raised concerns and made protected disclosures; if it has been effective, the persecution of whistleblowers would have stopped, but that has not happened – whistleblowers are still being persecuted.

The reason why the *Freedom To Speak Up Guardian* model does not work is because it suffers from the same underlying problem that the PIDA has, inasmuch that the responsibility for protecting a whistleblower lies with the whistlelower's employer which, typically, is the hospital or clinic that the whistleblower is complaining about. If the hospital (or clinic etc) wants some "bad news" buried, then the managers and directors are not going to be enthusiastic about an employee who opposes and threatens whatever issues they want suppressed. Neither are the managers and directors going to appoint *Freedom To Speak Up Guardians* who escalate concerns that employees bring to their attention. If the Guardians do what they are supposed to do, and ensure resolution of the concerns they are presented with, they will suffer the same retribution that the original whistleblowers experience; after all, the *Freedom To Speak Up Guardians* are also hospital employees, and their careers are as dependent on supporting the NHS cover-up culture as every other employee's career is.

♨ NHS Whistleblowers

If you, the reader, are an NHS employee who is contemplating raising a concern with a *Freedom To Speak Up Guardian*, there are two things that are worth considering:

♟ *Freedom To Speak Up Guardians* were introduced because the Public Interest Disclosure Act (PIDA) has proved to offer no protection to whistleblowers. If a whistleblower is not protected by a law that was specifically designed to protect them, it is reasonable to assume that another employee, who has been appointed a *Freedom To Speak Up Guardian*, does not have the will or authority to provide the protection that the PIDA is meant to provide.

☠ Why has your designated *Feeedom to Speak up Guardian* been appointed to that role? Would management appoint them because they are most likely to act in the interests of the public, and the whistleblower, by escalating and propagating the relevant issue? Or have they been appointed because they are more likely to be loyal to the cover-up culture, and protect the reputation of the hospital and its managers and directors?

What every NHS employee should know is that *Freedom To Speak Up Guardians* act as Quislings against them, and their perverted existence is only to protect their Chief Executives, the public image of the NHS, and the government of the day

In the NHS, nobody has the freedom to speak up!

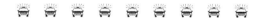

🚑 25: UNIONS

Trade unions, in the U.K., came into existence to counter the age old servant/master relationship between the poor and their ruling employers. Neither workers or the unemployed had rights of any kind, and life, for the masses, was one of hardship, disease, and suffering. Individually, these people had no power to improve their situations so, instinctively, they used the power of numbers to demand better working and living conditions, and first made their collective voice heard in the Luddite protests of 1812, culminating, eventually, in government acceptance of the union movement, with the Trade Union Act of 1871.

It is the union movement which can be thanked for continued improvements in worker safety and welfare and, without the unions, many people would not be alive today, because their ancestors would have died of industrial accidents or malnutrition.

In some areas of industry, and with some unions, progress is still being made to improve worker protection and welfare, but this is not true in the NHS, where union strength is diluted by too many competing unions and, depressingly, union corruption. By example, I will present the situation at that bastion of corruption - hospital T.

Union X

At hospital T, there are five active unions, all of whom compete for staff membership. The biggest union (X) has the support of management, and all new staff are encouraged to join this union.

Staff Induction

In the first week of employment, staff take part in an induction process, which consists of explanations of administrative tasks to be completed, such as obtaining identity cards and computer access, and listening to talks about what a wonderful place hospital T is.

Part of the induction phase is an introduction to union X, and its leader, Janet Pogrom, who spends an hour or so convincing the newcomers to join the union, because of the protection it gives them. One form of protection is in regard to the legal assistance the union provides to anyone who needs it. The thought of experiencing legal action is very worrying for staff, because all staff are aware of the scapegoating and blame culture of the NHS, so being protected by a firm of lawyers is a great comfort. It is because of this legal protection, more than anything else, which convinces new staff to join union X, and Janet Pogrom takes advantage of their fear by persuading them to join the union there and then – before they have the chance to join another union.

What Janet does not tell the new union members is that legal assistance is not automatic – it will only be approved if the union believes that the chances of winning the employee's case are greater than 95%. But, if winning their case is such a sure thing, the union member would not need legal assistance, so there would be no need of union help. Conversely, if the chances of winning were estimated to be less than 95%, the employee would not receive any legal assistance, they would have to face lawyers, representing the hospital, on their own, and they would be overwhelmed with legal clout, so would have little possibility of winning their case.

In summary, the union will supply legal help when the employee does not need it, but will deny legal help when the employee does need it. By all appearances, union X wants to use the winning of an easy legal case, which comes at no cost to them, to promote the benefits of joining the union to other employees, which means that legal help is designed to benefit the union – not the employee.

Why Union X?

The fact that hospital T grants union X sole representation at staff inductions seems suspicious, and for good reason. The union or, more specifically, Janet Pogrom, has no loyalty to union members, and will always take the side of the hospital in any dispute between union members and management. The motivation that Janet has for working against her union members is based on the very comfortable position she has, and which is maintained by her "Quisling" behaviour, in favour of management.

Janet Pogrom, Union Leader

Janet is employed as a nurse, and is allowed one day a week to devote to union duties. She does not work weekends, bank holidays, or night shifts, and she does not have to request holiday periods, as other nurses do – she takes them when she wants.

In reality, Janet does not perform any nursing related duties, and she is allowed to devote all of her time to union activities. She keeps her own hours, is not accountable for her schedule and, as long as she is present for disciplinary Hearings, does whatever she wants.

The members of union X do not become aware of Janet's treachery to them, until they need her help when, for example, they are being unfairly disciplined, or are suffering any type of discrimination or bullying. When staff need Janet's help, she interviews them about their case, and discerns what actions they might consider, when planning their defence. Once armed with the union member's confidential information, Janet passes it on to the personnel department chief "prosecutor", Alfred Neuman, who reacts accordingly, by plotting, with Janet, a plan of action which best deals with the union member.

If the union member's disciplinary case was initiated because a senior person, such as their manager, wants to be rid of the employee, Janet's instruction from Alfred will be to tell the employee that the case against them is very strong, will almost certainly end in punishment, and the consequences will be damaging to their career. Janet will then boast, to the union member, that she has used her influence and skill to persuade Alfred Neuman to allow the union member to avoid disciplinary action, by submitting his or her notice to leave the employ of the hospital.

Unions have come a long way since the days of the Luddites!

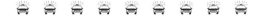

26: MODERN SLAVERY

Many nurses and allied health professionals (AHPs) are attracted to their professions because of the appeal produced by official government advertising and promotion of working in the medical field. To use nursing as an example, because everyone understands what a nurse is, advertisers make various promotional claims such as "Nursing is the most employable career in the UK", or "You will make a positive difference to people's lives", and "the opportunity to travel". It all sounds very exciting!

Nurse Training

Qualifying as a nurse (or AHP) involves a three year commitment to training, and a university loan to take out, for native staff. Once qualified, the average nurse is committed to a nursing career, and has to fit in with the NHS cover-up culture which, as they invariably discover, is surprisingly unpleasant. Together with the effects of being worried about paying off a loan, the reality of working in the NHS imposes a great stress on the new nurse or AHP.

As a consequence of their financial debt, and awareness that changing careers is impractical, many nurses become trapped in their new lives, and feel that they have lost much of their freedom, due to their forced compliance with the cover-up culture they are immersed in. Additionally, the inability to raise concerns, due to the constant deterrent threat of disciplinary action, makes nurses feel that their lives are controlled by their employer, and their freedom of expression is permanently curtailed.

🚑 Slavery

Slavery is a term which most people associate with the buying and selling of humans, in the history book styles recorded from pre Roman times, through to the nineteenth century when, in the western world at least, buying and selling of humans was abolished. Slavery has persisted, to this day, in many parts of the world and, in its various guises, has also been reintroduced into the United Kingdom and identified, more recently, by the umbrella term of "modern slavery". One definition of modern slavery, as provided by the ***anti-slavery*** organisation, is given as a person:

> "Trapped and controlled by an employer, by mental abuse or threat of mental abuse, and suffering criticism and disciplinary threats."

This definition of modern slavery intersects with the entrapment and threats of disciplinary action experienced by nurses and allied professionals. For those readers who have not worked in the NHS, associating modern slavery with being a nurse or AHP may seem an exaggeration but, you have to experience it to understand it.

🚑 27: PROFESSIONALISM

In order to portray the realities of how the NHS is staffed, it is necessary to describe the attitudes and behaviours, which some staff have, with regard to their professional and moral obligations towards patient care. In most cases, nurses, AHPs (allied health professionals), and other staff do act properly, and will always do whatever is necessary for the welfare of patients. There are, unfortunately, clinical professionals who do not comply with the standards of behaviour and professionalism which the public expect of them. These people might best be described as "rogues".

When any of these rogues is the cause of suffering, including the murder of patients, and there is widespread press reporting of those events, they are brought to book for what they have done.

Well known examples of rogue clinical professionals include Dr Harold Shipman, Dr Jane Barton, Dr Ian Paterson, Nurse Beverley Allitt, and Nurse Victorino Chua.

For less extreme examples of rogues, who do not habitually behave in the proper and professional manner that is expected of them, the situation is much different, because these people, and their behaviours, often "fly under the radar" of scrutiny, and are unsafe as much for what they **do not do**, as what they actually do. This is something which is best exemplified, by recounting an incident concerning, yet again, the senior anaesthetic technician (ODP) Albert Steptoe, during a Friday operating theatre department shift, when I witnessed a true representation of his attitude to the clinical job he is well paid to do.

Dangerous Team Leader

It was just before three p.m., when I had to retrieve an equipment carousel, which was stored in the main reseption area, and where the team leader offices were also located. As I was assembling the parts I needed, the department's main doors opened, and I saw several ICU (Intensive Care Unit) nurses, two anaesthetists and an anaesthetic technician, bring in a bed with an unconscious patient, who needed immediate and life-saving surgical intervention, in the emergency operating theatre, known as CEPOD (Confidential Enquiry into Perioperative Deaths). In such emergency cases, time is of the escence, and the patient has to be wheeled straight into the emergency operating theatre, transferred onto the operating table, and surgery commenced immediately. In parallel with surgery, the anaesthetist(s) have to keep the patient alive, ensuring their lungs are adequately ventilated (oxygen in, carbon dioxide out), and providing the patient with adequate volume and circulation of the circulatory system, applying appropriate drug administration regimes, and using various techniques and items of equipment to monitor and manage the patient's changing physiological condition. Anaesthetic assistants, either anaesthetic technicians or anaesthetic trained nurses, help anaesthetists by gathering and preparing whatever equipment might be needed, including rapid fluid infusion devices, invasive monitors, blood products, and other such specialist devices and resources.

To ensure all members of the emergency team are suitably employed in the above tasks of retrieving or setting up equipment, it is useful to have a team leader present, so that the team has proper coordination and communication, and the possibility of confusion or duplicating tasks is reduced. This is exactly what a band seven team leader is supposed to do – to lead the team.

Simultaneously with the ICU bed coming through the department doors, the anaesthetic team leader, Albert Steptoe, opened his office door and was backing out of the office whilst talking to his friend and ally, the anaesthetic team clinical practice educator, who I refer to as Paul Gadd. When Albert turned to close the door, he saw the ICU bed, and all of the commotion involved with managing the dying patient, especially the two anaesthetists ventilating (breathing for) the patient. Albert immediately reversed the closing motion of the door, and stepped back inside his office. One of the porters, who was holding open the door for the ICU bed, called my attention with "John!" I glanced over to him, and he mouthed "Did you see that?" I nodded my head in confirmation – I was too shocked by Albert's behaviour to answer in any other way. (I still am shocked)

As a team leader, Albert's job was to join the CEPOD team, quickly assess the situation, decide and prioritise the tasks to be performed, allocate and monitor those tasks, communicate with the anaesthetists, and use his authority and experience to coordinate whatever was necessary to produce a positive end result for the patient. Albert was not concerned about the patient; it was Friday afternoon, and his team's social events manager, Claire Middier, had organised his team's Friday night social session at an upmarket London pub, and two of the new young blondes were going to be present, which was a very exciting prospect for Albert, so he wanted to get away even earlier than he usually does, so that he would be as fresh as possible to receive his new girls – he did not want any distractions, and if the ICU patient died, what did he care?

An hour or so after this event, the porter who had earlier called over to me, informed me that Albert waited in his office for less than a minute after the ICU bed was pushed into the emergency theatre, before making his escape to another part of the hospital, where he changed into his street clothes, and slithered (his term) home. It was shortly after this event that I discovered that Albert has a long standing cocaine habit, which might explain his detachment from the reality of his position.

28: AGENCY WORKERS

The NHS has a policy of allowing flexible work hours for those who want to make specific arrangements which fit in with their personal commitments, particularly with respect to child care. However, this policy is another instance of propaganda, designed to make working in the NHS seem an appealing prospect. In practice, flexible working is reserved for senior or favoured staff. Moreover, denying flexible working hours to an employee is one of the methods that a manager uses to "encourage" a non-favoured worker to seek alternative employment.

For others, the problem of having to work inconvenient and antisocial hours is solved by leaving permanent employment, and taking up agency work, where there are no mandatory work times to be worked. Agency staff also have the benefit of avoiding the politics and cliqueyness which permeate the NHS. These two benefits of agency work are counter-balanced by lack of job security and, more significantly, lack of basic rights – agency workers are treated with a great deal of disdain by the hospitals who engage their services, and are often subject to abuse and unfair treatment, even though agency workers are meant to be protected by official *NHS Workers Regulations*. In addition to being treated as an under-class, agency workers are cheated, by the NHS, in a variety of ways, for example:

📖 Booking Shifts

When a hospital does not have someone to cover a particular shift, they will book an agency worker to fill that shift. Once booked, the hospital does not feel obliged to honour the shift, and they will continue to look for a permanent member of staff to fill the available shift through overtime (NHS term is "bank shift"). If the hospital is successful in finding a permanent member of staff to fill the shift, the agency worker will be informed, often at the last minute, that their shift has been cancelled, resulting in the agency worker losing a day's work, because it is too late for them to find a shift elsewhere. Sometimes, the agency worker will arrive at work, only to be told that they will not be needed. This is a tactic that a hospital uses so that, just in case a permanent member of staff phones in sick, at the last minute, the hospital has agency staff already on site, and the manager can choose amongst those people she (it usually is a she) wants to offer the shifts to. Those unselected agency staff will be compensated, for their cancelled booking, with two hours pay. The compensatory two hours pay may cover travel or parking expenses, but does not constitute real income. No other industry gets away with this practice of booking staff just in case they are needed, but the NHS gets away with it because the NHS is a government body and, like any other government body, it is all powerful and corrupt.

{The worst culprit hospitals of this unfair practice, in the London area are: Croydon, Hammersmith, **Royal Free**, Guys, **Kingston**, Royal London, **Northwick Park**, UCL, Epsom}

Coincidentally, <u>all</u> of these hospitals suffer persistent staff shortage problems, and they try to fix the shortfalls by bringing in a constant stream of nurses and anaesthetic technicians from poor countries, many of whom do NOT meet requirements for registration with the NMC or HCPC. What makes these people stand out is how they are often incapable of communicating or making a practical contribution when faced with emergency situations – they just make up the numbers, and they can be relied upon not to raise issues of concern - they are complicit in, and rely on, the NHS cover-up culture.

Some hospitals, such as Royal Free and Northwick Park, extend their abusive treatment of agency workers by failing to honour their legal obligation to pay the compensatory two hour cancellation fee, using the threat that, if the agency worker insists on being paid, they will be black-listed from further work at the hospital.

♨ Dishonesty

Not all hospital shifts are for a full day's work; there are often single session clinics and operating theatre lists which are only of a four hour duration. Agency staff do not get paid enough to do regular half day shifts (thank you, George Osborne), so an agency worker will usually only book a half day shift if there are no full day shifts available. Hospitals know that it is much more difficult to find cover for a half day, rather than a full day shift, so they will book an agency worker for a full day shift, but only give them a half day's work (worst culprits: Hammersmith, Guys and Royal London). This is dishonest and abusive behaviour for anyone hoping for an honest day's work. Two consequences of dishonestly treating agency staff in this, and other ways, include:

① A hospital with a reputation for playing this fake *full day booking* trick results in an increased probability of not attracting agency staff to fill vacant shifts, so causing elective (non-emergency) surgical lists to be cancelled, resulting in inconvenience to patients, and extra costs to the hospital (taxpayers).

② By tricking agency staff into working half day shifts, the hospital develops a reputation for abusive and dishonest behaviour towards agency staff, which quickly spreads, so the hospital has to rely on a constant stream of agency "new faces", all of whom are unfamiliar with the intricacies of how the particular department works, where equipment is stored, how to use the computer systems, how to get emergency blood components (without a security pass), and so on. Such unfamiliarity reduces productivity, increases risk to patients, and is a source of common complaint from the doctors who constantly have to work with people who they are unfamiliar with and, frequently, are unable to communicate with.

⚉ Underpaying

One issue, which many readers might consider to be of a trivial nature, but is symptomatic of the way agency workers are treated, is the common practice of deducting pay for rest and meal breaks, which the agency worker did not have. One establishment, Croydon hospital, is infamous for this practice. This always happens for one particular 8 a.m. to 2 p.m. shift, where the worker has to work the full six hours, without being relieved for either a ten minute tea break, or a half hour lunch break, but only gets paid for five and a half hours because, according to the manager, they should have taken these breaks. As anyone working in a clinical setting (ward, ICU etc) will confirm, if someone takes a break from their healthcare responsibilities, they can only do so if they have been officially relieved by someone else – they cannot just abandon their patients, so the management assertion that the worker should have taken a break would be unsafe practice. This is another NHS dirty trick which victims have to suffer and, if they make any sort of complaint, formally or not, they will be punished.

Being cheated out of a half hour's pay, some might say is not worth bothering about. However, if this happens every week, or every day, over a forty year career, the loss of income might be equivalent to losing one year's pay. It should also be borne in mind that this type of abusive behaviour increases the bad will felt by workers, and that decreases reliability – agency staff not turning up is not uncommon.

This small, but highly relevant matter, highlights the attitude of NHS clinical leaders to their principles of clinical leadership, which are supposed to generate good staff relations, rather than create adversarial feelings. Clinical leaders do not comply with their own leadership principles and, as a result, NHS managers create the very staff shortages which makes their jobs more difficult, and which they like to complain about.

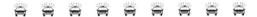

🚑 29: SAFE STAFFING LEVELS

The Francis investigation (2013) into the failings of Stafford Hospital, part of the Mid Staffordshire Hospital Trust, found that, in the period 2005 to 2009, between four and twelve hundred patients died, because of the poor care they were subject to. The main failings being reported as:

① Inadequate numbers of properly qualified and competent clinical staff, specifically nurses and allied professionals.

② Standards of hygiene were **non-existent**; patients would go for months without being washed, and had no assistance in toileting, so they would soil themselves in their beds.

③ Food and drinks were placed out of reach of infirm patients, so they would go without sustenance.

④ Patients were prematurely discharged (to meet targets); some of whom died as a result, and others had to be readmitted.

⑤ Non clinical staff were expected to assess and prioritise patients.

⑥ There was a toxic culture of bullying and threats by senior staff, against nurses, which discouraged them from speaking out.

The issue of safe staffing levels, the subject of this chapter, attracts much national publicity, and the NHS puts much effort into painting over the cracks, with various tricks and sleights of hand to make it appear that improvements are being made. Ministers, for example, will publish positive news, in social media, about increased staff numbers. However, since the Francis Report, researchers have discovered that no substantial improvements, across the NHS, have been made into ensuring safe staffing levels, and no steps have been taken to address the reasons for the shortage of numbers of suitably competent staff.

A University of Southampton report found that the Mid Staffs scandal has failed to prompt proper investment into nurse training and retention, and an increasing number of nurses are being substituted with unqualified staff. The University of Southampton also discovered that, for every twenty-five patients, replacing a nurse with a lower qualified employee resulted in a twenty-one percent increase in patient deaths.

📠 Fake Nurses

An example of this problem of substituting qualified with unqualified staff, is that of the growing tendency for hospitals to give on-the-job training to healthcare assistants, supported by courses (with no substance) at universities, to make them appear "qualified" to do the work that nurses and anaesthetic technicians would normally do. The advantage to the hospitals is the dependency which these pseudo qualified staff have on being employed in better paid posts than they would otherwise be, and that dependency is accompanied by their loyalty to the NHS cover-up culture, which means more security for management. What this practice of fiddling with professional qualifications does not do is increase standards of care, neither does it meet the requirements of the Health and Safety at Work Act (HASAW) to reduce risk and, because of that, it contravenes the Act, which is a criminal offence.

▨ Safe, Sustainable and Productive Staffing

To meet the recommended safe numbers of staff, guidelines have been produced by *NHS Improvement*, on behalf of the NHS *National Quality Board*, under the subject title "Safe, Sustainable and Productive Staffing". What is notable about these guidelines is that they explicitly declare that their intention is to ensure that NHS Providers (hospitals etc) **"deliver the right staff, with the right skills, in the right place, and at the right time"**, and that safe staffing levels include an "uplift" of staff numbers, which means extra staff to cover absences, such as sickness and leave periods.

To satisfy the public that safe staffing numbers are being maintained, the government have incorporated staffing levels into the target culture of the NHS. Hospital wards/departments are mandated to record the daily required staff numbers against actual numbers, and report those numbers to senior managers and directors. Notably, the decision about staff levels is subjectively and dynamically made by ward matrons and managers, and those numbers can change throughout the shift. The recorded figures are usually posted at the entrance to wards, because they are propaganda for public consumption.

The problem with this practice is that there is no assurance of veracity, so ward managers and matrons can post whatever information they want the public to see, and can change those numbers to suit expectations, which is that required staff numbers match actual numbers. The public have no opportunity to verify that the posted figures are correct, and ward or departmental managers and matrons do not want to attract negative attention from senior management, so the opportunity to mislead is obvious and, irresistable. For example, if the department or ward needs twenty employees, but only fifteen are present, the publicly posted (usually at the department entrance) numbers can show that fifteen staff are needed, and fifteen staff are present, which means there is a safe staffing level. If two more staff arrive, during that shift, the posted numbers can be changed to show seventeen staff are needed, and seventeen staff are present, and so on.

The number of staff on duty is not the only thing that can be manipulated, because there is also the issue of what type of staff members are being reported in official figures for safe staffing levels. For example, if a particular ward needs eight nurses to satisfy the ward's pre-determined safe staffing level, and there are, indeed, eight staff members on duty, it is possible that one or more (possibly all) of those nurses are not nurses at all – they might be healthcare assistants who have become "fake nurses". In this instance, the numbers meet the required target, in terms of what is recorded, but not in terms of qualifications for the job in hand, because fake nurses do not have to meet any professional or registration requirements to deliver safe healthcare services.

There is no mechanism to prevent this type of manipulation of figures. Incidentally, external bodies, such as the CQC, are unlikely to catch this problem, because their arrival in hospital is always known in advance, so there is plenty of opportunity to bring in extra agency staff to meet the safe staff number target for the duration of the CQC's inspection.

For the particular ward or departmental manager, who reports the figures for staffing levels, the pressure on them can be overbearing; if they report an unsafe staffing level as being safe, they will satisfy the standard requirements of the NHS cover-up culture, and their job will not be under threat; conversely, if they accurately report that the department or ward has an inadequate number of staff, then that information gets fed, ultimately, to the Department of Health. Such information, which enters the public domain, reflects badly on the government, and their image with the public can be jeopardised. Pressure, then, is brought to bear on that hospital's Chief Executive, who will not be too pleased that his/her Medical or Nursing Director has not ensured the "right" figures have been reported.

In the NHS, pressure and blame flow down the chain of command, and it will be the departmental manager, responsible for generating the unsafe staffing figure, who will suffer, either through the bullying tactic of implied threats of demotion, or the inferred threat of a negative gossip campaign of incompetence against them. Whatever method is used, the departmental manager is in a catch-22 situation – they cannot win.

⚱ Having the Right Staff

A significant fault in having a safe staff level target is the lack of consideration of who the staff are, because there is no practical emphasis on ensuring the right type of staff, with respect to their abilities, social and communication skills, or suitability for their roles. This is why the NHS employs people who are fraudulently qualified, or cannot express themselves in English. The target is quantity – not quality, or safety.

Fake Staff and Discrimination

A particularly noticeable problem, with respect to the NHS

employing so many poorly and fraudulently qualified staff, is that of the defensive attitude those fraudsters have against staff members who are properly competent and qualified, especially when the fake staff form a majority in the department. To protect their positions, the fraudsters put much effort in making the employment experiences for the genuinely competent staff as unpleasant as they can, and make it clear that they do not want to establish any sort of normal teamwork relationship with them; the fake professionals do not want anyone asking them anything about their training, or their abilities. The reason for this is that the fraudsters do not want properly qualified staff members to be around long enough to discover the inadequacies and "secrets" of these unqualified people, and they do not want the qualified staff members to remain long enough to stand out as being more knowledgeable and competent than the fraudsters, because that could focus negative attention onto the fraudsters. By successfully establishing a virtual "fraudsters only" employment policy, the fraudsters are able to build up their power bases, through seniority, because departmental promotion is mostly limited to the people already in the respective teams.

The safety implications of these centres of power, for the fraudsters, become most apparent when an emergency arises, because the fraudsters do not like to get involved in dealing with whatever emergency they are confronted with which, typically, is an airway or cardiac problem. During such times, the arrogance and antisocial behaviours of the "fakes" changes to friendly requests for assistance from properly qualified staff, in dealing with the emergency, accompanied by temporary suspensions of their antisocial attitudes towards those genuine practitioners.

* * *

So, for a particular clinical department, there may appear to be a safe staffing level, in regard to numbers, but not for the quality or competency of staff, which is something that is never measured, but is universally covered-up, as per the culture of the NHS.

♦ Victorino Chua

There can be no better example of how the NHS emphasises staff quantity over quality, than that of nurse Victorino Chua, who murdered several English patients, at his place of work, Stepping Hill Hospital, (Stockport), in 2015.

Chua killed his victims by sabotaging their intravenous fluids with deadly levels of insulin, and tried to blame English nurses for his crimes. Chua took pleasure from seeing his patients die, and from witnessing the shock and stress invoked on those nurses who were, initially, held accountable for his actions. Chua described himself as "evil", and claimed the devil was inside him, and he expressed no remorse for his crimes.

As part of the criminal case against Chua, police discovered that his nurse qualifications were fake. The prosecuting lawyer, Nazir Afzal, reported that it was extremely worrying that "many untrained and unqualified foreign workers are working in UK hospitals". The uncovering of Chua's "qualifications" prompted a BBC investigation, which found that Chua bought his nursing qualification, in the Phillipines, for thirty US dollars, from Recto University (see later).

To work as a nurse, in the UK, the nurse has to register with the Nursing and Midwifery Council (NMC), whose official function is to "protect the health and wellbeing of the British public". By accepting a nurse onto their register, the NMC is giving the assurance, to the public, that the newly registered nurse can safely provide nursing care. The NMC, however, do not screen nurses for validity of their knowledge and abilities, and they do not verify the authenticity of their paper qualifications. If they were committed to protecting the public, the NMC could have commissioned some basic research to learn how easy, or not, it would be to obtain fraudulent qualifications in foreign countries, such as is the case in the Philippines – if the BBC can do it, then so can the NMC. Armed with such knowledge about fraudulent qualifications, the NMC would be better prepared to put a system in place that would properly filter out those frauds. In so doing, the NMC would be satisfying their mission statement "protect the health and wellbeing of the British public".

♣ Nursing and Midwifery Council (NMC)

Acceptance onto the NMC register is mostly a tick box exercise, which serves to increase the "nursing numbers", in line with the government staff level targets (annual registration subscriptions also help fill the NMC coffers). If the NMC employed a proper verification system, which filtered out unsuitable or unqualified applicants, nurse Chua would not have been accepted onto the NMC register, and he would not have had the opportunity to murder his victims. The NMC might say that a proper verification system would not be feasible, because it would be too time consuming and expensive to run, but filtering out the likes of Chua is what the NMC exists to do, so it is their job to find a solution to any difficulties they anticipate. If cost is considered a primary obstruction to proper screening, applicants for registration can pay for the screening system themselves, after all, they are the ones who benefit from employment with the NHS. There is nothing wrong with that idea, in fact, such a system would deter many of the fraudsters from making applications, because they would know that failing to pass an acceptance test would cost them their testing fee, so they would not bother to apply in the first place. With the current system, there is no risk to being rejected by the NMC.

If the NMC want to continue giving numbers of nurses priority over validity of their qualifications, then the NMC has no value, serves no proactive purpose, and should be disbanded.

The NMC is NOT fit for purpose.

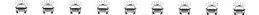

⛟ 30: CAREER DETERRENTS

T here are a number of reasons for the persistent NHS problem of inadequate numbers, abilities, and experience of staff, particularly nurses and allied health professionals (AHPs). Using nursing as an example (because everyone understands their role), some of the principle reasons of shortages include:

⚱ Low Pay

According to the UK government's own classification system, nursing is a "low paid" vocation. For some people who might otherwise be attracted to the profession, the low pay factor is one that can serve as a serious deterrent, especially because of its life style consequences. Career choice factors can be exemplified by:

1. One where remuneration leads to affording only a small terraced house, in a poor area, with schools where the children are at risk of violence, and where drug use is the norm.

2. One that is more likely to lead to owning a larger and detached house, in a respectable neighbourhood, and where private education is attainable and affordable.

Option "1" is the more likely outcome for nurses and AHPs, so is a significant career deterrent.

♣ Training Fees

Since free training for most British nurses (and AHPs) was abolished, the millstone of paying back education loans, for such low paid careers, has made them even worse career choices, especially as the training is very narrow and specific to a career with non-transferrable skills.

♣ Registration Dependency

If someone chooses to train as, for example, a geologist, chef, or bookkeeper, they will work within their chosen field without having to be constantly at the acquiescence of their employer's cultural beliefs (cover-up culture etc), and without having to persistently satisfy their registration body (GMC, NMC, HCPC) that they publicly support the existence and function of that body; if, for example, a registrant were to criticise their registration body, that body would deem the registrant as acting against the general interests of their profession and, consequently, would remove the registrants membership, and their right to continue working in that profession. Similarly, if the registrant's employer wanted to punish the registrant for some transgression (e.g. whistleblowing), they would find "good" reason to report the employee to their registration body, who would then suspend or remove the employee's registration.

It is because of the registration body requirement that so few registrants (nurses etc) feel free to speak out about issues of public concern – they know that the retribution process will lead to loss of registration, so they have to "toe the line", and not do anything to show the NHS, or the government, in a bad light. Registration bodies serve to deter registrants from raising issues that might reflect poorly on the government, who they exist to protect, rather than serving the public, who they are supposed to protect.

For the privilege, and the Sword of Damocles hanging over them, of having a registration body deciding whether or not a healthcare worker should be allowed to continue in their career, registrants have to pay annual subscriptions to those bodies, and with nothing positive, such as protection from retribution for whistleblowing or bullying and discrimination, in return. Of course, registration bodies will claim that they act in the interests of public safety, by ensuring that convicted felons are not allowed on their professional registers, but such prohibitions could be easily enforced by legal means, so registration bodies are redundant, because they do nothing to protect the public, and that is why there are so many unsuitable people working in the NHS.

As mentioned in the chapter on MODERN SLAVERY, being trapped in a job, where employment is dependent on confirming to behaviours which may be illegal or immoral, and where there is no real freedom to raise concerns, without suffering punishment for doing so, meets with the definition of modern slavery. This is not the case for the likes of the previously mentioned bookkeepers, geologists, chefs, and so on, whose job security is only dependent on doing their jobs properly - these people are not at the mercy of registration bodies, and they do not have to pay registration fees for the privilege of being allowed to work, neither do they have to conform with their employer's unwritten beliefs or public propaganda schemes, which is the case with NHS employment.

♠ Unsocial Lifestyle

Working in a hospital, for clinical staff – not managers and directors – means living an unhealthy and anti-social lifestyle. If the low pay and inequalities are not a deterrent, then the prospect of switching between day and night shifts, working weekends, and being available for twenty-four hour "on-call" rotas should be, especially as various researchers (Princeton and Surrey Universities, 2018) have proved that these constantly changing work patterns reduce life expectancy, and increase the probability of: **stroke, heart attack, breast cancer, accidents, depression, obesity, and diabetes**. *The World Health Organisation* (2017) also report that the change in circadian rhythms, caused by night shifts, increases the risk of developing **all** types of cancer. A similar report, by the *International Agency for Research on Cancer* (2019) declares that night shift working is carcinogenic to humans. Predictably, NHS hospitals do not warn staff of the above threats to their health that anti-social working hours produce – they prefer to keep such things secret.

♠ Yob Culture

Television shows like to portray NHS clinical workers as cooperative, collegiate, respectful, and professional. At times, this can be a true reflection of the work environment culture. Generally, the reality is very different, because the working environment is better described by behaviours that are anti-social, uncooperative, discriminatory, disrespectful, and polluted with bullying, aggression, inequalities, jealousies, and favouritism. These behaviours are ubiquitous and relentless in the NHS, and only differ between hospitals or departments, by the degree to which they are encouraged or tolerated by managers, many of whom are very divisive characters, who thrive on making tactical staff alliances, and practicing favouritism, all with the aim of protecting their positions.

The yob culture, in the NHS, does not make for a happy workplace but, instead, puts people constantly on their guard against sabotage, bitchiness, and back-stabbing. These things, of course, are in opposition to a team spirit atmosphere that would allow employees to concentrate on their work, and protect them from distractions, so they may better focus on their jobs. The yob culture makes the NHS an unappealing employer, and is one of the holes in the *Swiss Cheese* model of safety (Health & Safety Executive) that make failures more likely. Notably, this issue of yobbishness is never raised by anyone at any level in the NHS; it is another thing unspoken by employees, and kept secret from the public.

♣ Peer Jealousy and Career Sabotage

The NHS is not a meritocracy. Career development is dependent on departmental managers, to those who are either of a favoured status (including hanky-panky relationships), or who pose the least threat to the manager's position and status. Those who do have the potential to reach advanced and senior positions, are subject to jealousies by their less able peers, who often try to make their more capable colleagues seem inadequate, either in a professional sense, or in terms of their personal and social skills. Spreading malicious gossip is probably the most popular method of sabotaging the career prospects of these more competent workers, and that is because it is the most successful one. The NHS society is so filled with jealousies and cliquishness, that people will willingly go along with derogatory gossip about a colleague, who they think may be heading for promotion, or may have "raised concerns", in the hope that the gossip campaign will halt that promotion.

Career sabotage also occurs when a group of employees from one particular country want to stop someone, who is foreign to them, from achieving seniority over them, in the hope that one of their own group gets the job instead. The reason for this is because there are so many unsafe NHS employees who either have fake qualifications, or who lack the ability that is demanded by their roles, that having a team leader or manager who is from the same country as them, gives them a level of protection; they have symbiotic relationships, so "outsiders" are not welcome. This "closed shop" behaviour, incidentally, is another reason for high staff turnover – people do not stay where they are unwelcome.

♣ Discrimination, Favouritism, Bullying

These are probably the most significant factors that make employment in the NHS so unattractive and, for anyone lucky enough to be aware of these anti-social and anti-functional cultures, avoiding a career in healthcare is a wise step.

♣ Complying with the NHS Cover-up Culture

Another poorly kept "secret" of working in the NHS is the requirement that the cover-up culture has to be respected and maintained. Anyone who does not comply with this unspoken imperative will face a tortuous bullying campaign that will either force them into compliance, or will force them out of their profession. In either case, the accumulated mental stress that they experience will adversely affect their health and wellbeing.

Unfortunately, many prospective entrants into healthcare professions are either unaware of these most negative aspects of their chosen careers, or are warned about them, but dismiss them as issues that affect other people – they have the attitude that bullying and other unfair treatments will not happen to them. They only change their minds once they have been immersed into the blame and cover-up culture of the NHS. That is probably why so many people have short careers in the NHS.

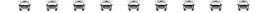

31: ATTEMPTED MURDER OF A NURSE

There is frequent and well known public debate about the continued survival of the NHS, and the potential of it being subsumed into the private sector. It is unlikely that any government would allow such a thing to happen, because it would be a major vote losing action. However, what may not be so well known, to the general public, is that NHS hospitals already operate in the private sector, and do so to boost there incomes, by undertaking private surgical cases. If taking private cases is of financial benefit to a hospital, the question must be asked "Do NHS patients take priority, or does the extra income from the private sector mean the priority is tilted towards those money making private cases?". The definitive answer to that question can only be answered by INDEPENDENT forensic auditing of the hospitals concerned.

However, a relatively recent (2019) incident helps shine some light on this issue of conflicting interests between the NHS and the private sector. Specifically, the incident concerns a nurse who found herself a victim of attempted murder, after questioning why a private patient took priority over an NHS patient.

The Cardiac Patient

The incident started when the nurse was at her usual place of work, in the cardiac ward of St George's Hospital, Tooting. Her job was to make ready a bed and other facilities for an elderly patient, who was scheduled to be admitted for heart surgery. Prior to a patient having a major operation, a nurse has to make many preparations, to ensure that the patient is in a fit state to undergo anaesthesia. These preparations include ensuring equipment is available for physiological observations, administration of fluids and medications, and making various checks, such as ensuring the patient is properly fasted, has all allergies documented, and ensuring that paperwork is current. After this particular nurse had completed her preparations for her cardiac patient, she was instructed to visit the personnel department (I do not like the term "human resource") to tend to an administrative issue. When she returned to the ward, she was surprised to find a different patient, from the one expected, in the bed which she had recently prepared. Thinking that either there was a change of plan, or a mistake had been made, she asked her team leader, a senior nurse (band 7) to enlighten her of the situation. She (cardiac nurse) was told, in a hostile and unprofessional manner, to mind her own business and just do her job. This was quite a surprising reaction, and it left the nurse not a little confused about the aggressive reaction from her team leader but, familiar as she was with the bullying culture of the hospital, she did not take the matter further. What was clear was that the team leader wanted to deflect from the fact that the NHS patient had been "bumped" in favour of a private case, and this occurred in spite of the government's own assertion that:

"The United Kingdom government allocates public funds soley to NHS patients.", *Parliamentary policy paper, NHS Mandate, 2019.*

⚔ Disciplinary Action

Some days later, the nurse received notification, from the personnel department's lead bully, Alfred Neuman, that she was to face disciplinary action for her aggressive and uncooperative manner towards her team leader.

The nurse was doubly shocked at this; firstly, because of the false accusation and, secondly, because of the shame and stress that she knew she was about to suffer, due to the cruel and harsh reputation the hospital had for disciplining staff, and for always finding them guilty of whatever they were accused of.

In the NHS, when a senior person makes an accusation against a junior person, the personnel clerks will always take the side of the senior person, particularly in cases of active or potential whistleblowing.

The nurse decided to contest the case against her, and informed Alfred Neuman accordingly.

⚔ Death Threats

Some days later, the nurse received the first of several written death threats, sent via the hospital's internal mail system.

The manner of this death threat, itself, illustrates the level of clumsiness and stupidity of NHS management, because the use of the internal mail system means that the person making the threats has revealed that they work in the hospital.

After recovering from her initial shock, the nurse called the police, who took the letter for examination, and kept it as evidence. They (the police) then informed the hospital's security department that, should the nurse receive any more letters of this kind, someone from the hospital security team should don gloves, place the letter in a plastic bag, and leave it for the police to collect.

Subsequently, the nurse received three more letters, and these were collected by the security team. When the police arrived to retrieve the letters, they learnt that security staff had lost the letters. "Losing" a single might have been a mistake, but losing all three is very suspicious. It is quite apparent that the security staff were in collusion with whomever was making the death threats against the nurse. The combination of these lost letters, the death threats, and the disciplinary action against the nurse, were too overwhelming for her to continue working, so she signed off sick.

⚰ Attempted Murder

About one week after she went off sick, the nurse was awakened from a night's sleep, by the smell of burning. She went downstairs, and saw that a burning bundle of rags had been pushed through the letterbox of her front door. Immediately, she led her two sleeping children from the house, then called the fire brigade and police. After their initial investigations, the police installed various security cameras in and around the house, and opened a serious incident investigation.

After a six week period of sick leave, the personnel department (Alfred Neuman) informed the nurse that the hospital had imposed on her a six week limit for paid sick leave. With bills to pay, the nurse returned to work, even though she was in no frame of mind to do so.

Three weeks after resuming her duties, the nurse suffered another traumatic experience. On her way home from work, a man ran up behind her, and drop kicked her, in the middle of the back. After admitting herself to treatment for facial injuries, the nurse reported the incident to the police. She was now in real fear of her safety, and the prospect of returning to work was too dangerous and frightening for her, so she quit her job.

> The chapter on *Whistleblowers* describes another instance where arson has been used as a threat - nurse **Jennie Fecitt**.

🚌 Cover-up and Intimidation

The links between the death threats, the murder attempt, and physical assault are extremely unlikely to be coincidental, indeed, it would be unreasonable to think that they could have been. Additionally, it would be unreasonable to assume, or assert, that there could be no link between the threats and attempted murder, and the initial incident with a private paying patient given priority over an NHS patient.

This is all part and parcel of the corruption, fraud, bullying, and cover-up culture of the NHS and, referring to the original question about precedence between private and NHS patients, this case shows that private patients can, and do, take precedence over NHS patients. You, the reader, should make up your own mind about this matter but, before you do, consider the day, if it happens, when you, or a family member, have to undergo a major life saving operation; would you object to being pushed down a waiting list, so that your NHS hospital can make a wad of money from a private patient?

⚅ 32: FRAUD & WASTE

The NHS has a huge budget which, for the financial year of 2020-21 is £128 billion. With such a large amount of money, there is, inevitably, a significant amount of fraud and waste, with estimates for fraud alone being over one percent of the total budget. Much of the fraud, of course, especially minor cases, goes undetected, so the true figure is unknown. NHS fraud is such a significant problem, that the government introduced the Bribery Act, in 2011, to support the *NHS Digital* authority, which produces standards in regards to bribery, fraud, and corruption.

To address the fraud problem, specifically, the NHS has formed the *Counter Fraud Authority*, whose sole duty is to keep taxpayer's money from the clutches of crooks, both internal and external to the NHS. More in depth information about the work of the NHS Counter Fraud Authority, can be found at:

https://www.telegraph.co.uk/men/thinking-man/nhs-fraud-squad-catching-medical-insiders-stealing-13-billion/

The Counter Fraud Authority concentrates its resources on large scale and persistent cases of fraud, but it does not have the resources to detect or investigate cases which can be classed as relatively small. Neither does it have the necessary information which would enable it to conduct the more minor investigatory cases, primarily because that would mean relying on whistleblowers, and NHS employees know of the consequences to themselves, should they choose to become whistleblowers, so these people are few and far between. To illustrate how small scale fraud is realised, the following short exposé shows how easy it is for a corrupt NHS employee to abuse their power and privilege, for personal gain.

⛟ Overtime Fraud

NHS hospitals are always very busy, and rarely fully staffed. For some patients who must undergo surgery, there might not be available capacity to conduct their operations on week days, so they might be placed on an extra operating list, for a Saturday. Because there are not enough theatre staff to cover these extra weekend elective (non-emergency) lists, hospitals rely on staff to do overtime, which the NHS refer to as "bank" work. These weekend bank shifts are quite desirable to junior staff, because they pay a higher rate than during the week, and there are no team leaders (band seven) or managers (band eight) to harass them in the usual jobsworth manner these senior people thrive on. Band eight managers do not work at weekends, nights, or during public holidays, and team leaders (band seven) will only work on a Saturday if they want to do an easy and lucrative overtime shift, which they deny from junior staff.

A very good example of an anaesthetic technician team leader, who regularly works the Saturday overtime shift, is that of the repeat offender Albert Steptoe, at hospital T, who usually awards himself the Saturday shift - with a particular twist.

What makes anaesthetic technician Steptoe so noteworthy is that he does not just assign himself an easy Saturday shift, but he authorises his own timesheet, which usually means recording his work hours as 08:00 to 17:30, even though he rarely finishes after midday. Sometimes, his Saturday shift is for just one minor and simple surgical case, which takes less than one hour, but he still awards himself a full day's pay. He then slips away, undetected (he thinks), by leaving the theatre department in his "scrub" clothing, and changing into his own clothes, which are kept in another department. Albert makes several thousand pounds a year for these extra shifts, and has been doing so since the early 2000's.

The question that a taxpayer might ask is: "If it is so easy for this particular person to commit such an obvious fraud, then how many other NHS employees are defrauding the taxpayer, and in what other ways?".

⚙ Public Finance Initiative

PFI, as it is known, is the surreptitious entry of the private sector, into the NHS, which involves private sector financial investment, in return for lucrative returns. PFI is the mother lode of investment types - a high return for low risk.

When PFI was first introduced, in the early 1990s, it was very small scale, and had no noticeable effect on the public purse, However, with the late 1990s change of government, PFI escalated to a great degree, and has resulted in crippling debt for many hospitals, to the extent that they have to cut services so that they can service their debt on the private finance loans. Much more detailed information about PFI can be found on the internet but, for those readers who are unfamiliar with the subject, the following three examples of hospitals that have to waste money on servicing PFI debt, each year, might help to inform:

Coventry Trust: Pays £89 million p.a. on PFI debt.

Sherwood Forest Trust: Pays one sixth of its budget on PFI debt.

Barts Trust: Pays £116 million p.a. on PFI debt.

The money spent on servicing PFI debt is redirected from patient care and services, which means that NHS services are degraded, for the benefit of the private sector.

📣 Public Relations Spending

The NHS suffers from waste, just as much as it suffers from fraud, and spending on so called "public relations", which is propaganda by another name, is a significant misdirection of money that is intended for NHS patients. According to a BBC investigation in 2013, the NHS spent £13 million on public relations, which is enough money to pay for six hundred extra nurses. (What this figure is today is something which might be the subject of further investigation):

https://www.bbc.co.uk/news/uk-england-london-21762939

Spending millions of pounds on propaganda is of great benefit to NHS officials and the government, but is no benefit to patients.

🪴 Reasons for Public Relations Spending

The purpose of spending money on public relations (PR) is to enhance the image of the particular commissioning NHS entity, typically a hospital. The techniques used are very simple ones, the hospital produces pamphlets and web pages, complete with staged photographs of happy hospital employees and managers, with even happier patients, and all accompanied by success stories about how the hospital has enhanced the welfare of the featured patients. Ultimately, the PR propaganda is meant to enhance the standing of the Chief Executive and board of directors and, thereby, helps ensure they keep their seats on the NHS gravy train.

🚑 Legal Costs

♟ Reputation Management Spending

Another significant misdirection of taxpayer's money, away from patient care, and aimed at protecting NHS executives, is the use of corporate law firms to "mask" negative information about the hospital, and its mismanagement of the healthcare function. This combination of propaganda and maskirovka is known as "reputation management", and is a cause of significant drawing of funds from the annual healthcare budget.

By using expert legal counsel to protect their lucrative directorships, Chief Executives also, indirectly, protect the reputation of the government, so there is every motivation for politicians to encourage NHS hospitals to manage their reputations. Indeed, the NHS Confederation publish guidelines for hospitals to follow, entitled *Reputation management: a guide for boards*, which contains the following statement:

> NHS boards are increasingly recognising that the financial position of their organisations, whether they are a commissioner or provider, can be influenced significantly by their reputation.

The subtext of the above paragraph is:

If you fail cover-up any issue that might reflect badly on the government, then some of your funds will be withheld.

It is ironic that, even though these guidelines are intended to stimulate adherence to the NHS cover-up culture, no attempt has been made to cover-up the publication or distribution of the guidelines themselves – they are on the world wide web. Perhaps "they" thought nobody would notice?

A relatively recent example of NHS "reputation management" is the case of Great Ormond Street Hospital (GOSH), which awarded £130,000 to one law firm, Schillings, a specialist in "Managing Reputations" of wealthy clients. The law firm was commissioned to put a more positive sheen on a series of incidents where children experienced poor and dangerous care, whilst being treated at the hospital - as reported in the Guardian newspaper:

https://www.theguardian.com/society/2018/jul/24/great-ormond-street-childrens-hospital-spent-130000-on-reputation-management-lawyers

It is curious that no politicians take an interest in this type of waste of taxpayer's money, especially as it is something which taxpayers have no say in, and have no opportunity to express their feelings about. If the public were to question this misuse of public funds, one useful question might be "Who benefits from protecting a hospital's image, and who suffers for it?". We, the public, know the answer to that question, but it would be enlightening to be gifted with the answer from politicians.

♣ Punishment

NHS staff who have defended themselves in court (Employment Tribunals), against unfair disciplinary action, perhaps as punishment for whistleblowing, will be well aware of another unaccountable form of wasted money that is redirected from patient care, which is the spending a hospital makes to commission legal representation to defend the hospital against the disciplined employee's claim of unfair treatment or dismissal.

One law firm, in particular, which receives taxpayer money for helping ensure that punishment for NHS employees is upheld in Employment Tribunals, and protecting the reputation of hospitals, is *Capsticks Law*. A search on google, with terms such as "NHS Capsticks" will produce a list of web pages where Capsticks describe how they protect the good name of the NHS, by helping institutions, such as hospitals, with services to:

① Prepare for CQC (Care Quality Commission) investigations

② Problem solving

③ Manage employee relations

There are several questions that should be asked about how spending taxpayer's money on the above legal services helps the NHS in the provision of healthcare services. For example, how and why does a law firm help a hospital pass an inspection from the CQC, when the function of the CQC is to monitor, inspect, and regulate health and social care? Do lawyers know more about health and social care than doctors and nurses? "Problem solving" - what problems can a law firm solve for a hospital, and why would a hospital need legal help in solving problems? What are the hospitals doing so wrong that a law firm can dedicate itself to NHS problems? As for "Managing employee relations", that is just spin for the law firm representing the hospital when an employee has taken them to an Employment Tribunal for unfair dismissal. "Managing employee relations" does not include providing employees with legal services – the NHS is not a fair and equal employer, it will only allocate taxpayer money to attack employees, not to give them the same level of legal representation which the hospital uses against them.

To put this matter of waste into a more meaningful perspective, the NHS spent approximately £2 billion on legal fees in 2019. Some readers might suggest, to their members of parliament, better ways of spending that £2 billion; perhaps a new hospital - every year!

📧 Personal Relationships

The fraudulent promotion and other career development opportunities for some employees, as reward for having personal relationships with senior members of staff, is ubiquitous in the NHS, and is easily identified. In other industries, this is a matter that might not draw much attention, because it is part and parcel of human behaviour – it occurs everywhere. When this sort of reward for "personal services" occurs in the healthcare setting, it can compromise the duty to reduce risk to patients, because promotion is tied to greater responsibility for decision making and healthcare delivery and, because the promotion is not based on merit, the person being promoted may not be the best person to assume those greater responsibilities, or to make the best decisions to produce optimum patient outcomes. Additionally, when this situation happens, and it happens a lot, a more competent person, who is more deserving, will have been cheated out of the promotion. Interestingly, the Oxford English Dictionary definition of fraud coincides with what happens when a promotion is based on reward for a personal relationship: *"A person who pretends to have qualities or abilities that they do not really have, in order to cheat other people."*

🗐 Unpaid Shifts

There is an issue that occurs in some hospitals which, if not illegal, should be which, specifically, is the unofficial requirement that some locum doctors, who have applied for permanent employment at a hospital, are expected to complete unpaid shifts, before being considered for permanent employment. This is an issue that should be considered with respect to a definition of modern slavery: "A condition of having to work, without proper remuneration."

When, for example, an anaesthetist is assigned to an emergency operating theatre, with the job of keeping a patient alive (that is what they do), that patient's family might be distressed and shocked to learn that the person keeping their relative alive is a victim of modern slavery. It is more likely that they would prefer to think that the anaesthetist is being well paid for the job they do.

By failing to renumerate a doctor, a hospital gains a financial advantage, and a little further thought reveals an even larger advantage occurs, because the unpaid worker is extremely unlikely to report any wrongdoing – they are too desperate to blow the whistle, so they reinforce the hospital's cover-up culture.

This is another **dirty secret** that exposes how the NHS ignores the basic human rights of some of its most important workers.

32: WHISTLEBLOWING

The NHS Constitution includes an expectation that NHS staff will raise concerns as early as possible and a pledge that NHS employers will support all staff in raising concerns, responding to and where necessary investigating the concerns raised.

Whistleblowing is the popular term to describe the process of revealing, to an appropriate body, any matter which is being concealed, or covered up, that might be of public interest. The United Kingdom government defines *whistleblowing* as:

"The term used when a worker passes on information concerning wrongdoing, more formally known as 'making a disclosure' or 'blowing the whistle'. To meet the terms of being a disclosure, the whistleblower must believe that they are acting in the public interest, and the matter to which they refer concerns any one or more instance of fraud, safety, criminality, or failure to comply with legal statutes. Additionally, any case of covering up any disclosure is, itself, a disclosure that should be reported."

To satisfy their legal obligation to ensure the public interest is best served, employers are expected to create open, transparent, and safe working environments in which employees feel free to speak up or raise concerns about matters that meet the requirements for making disclosures. The phenomenon of using whistleblowing to counter something that is being concealed, or being covered up, is not uniquely a British one. Indeed, this is also a matter being addressed by the United States Government; Barack Obama accurately expressed the value of whistleblowing by employees of government organisations in his declaration: "Often, the best source of information about fraud and abuse in government is from government employees".

NHS Constitution, Staff Rights (part 4a)

"Staff can raise any concern with their employer, whether it is about safety, malpractice or other risk, in the public interest."

"The NHS commits to encourage and support all staff in raising concerns at the earliest reasonable opportunity about safety, malpractice or wrongdoing at work, responding to and, where necessary, investigating the concerns raised and acting consistently with the Employment Rights Act 1996 (pledge)."

Barriers to Raising Concerns

According to the Department for Business Innovation and Skills "Guidance and Code of Practice on Whistleblowing", employees face two barriers to making disclosures: firstly, no action will be taken as a result of the disclosure and, secondly, fear of reprisal for making the disclosure. Evidence to support these assertions of barriers to raising concerns, in the NHS, was most recently made public by the Lord Francis Mid Staffordshire Public Inquiry, and was published in Lord Francis's *Freedom to Speak Up* review (2014).

Health Service Safety Investigations Body

To counter the barriers to raising concerns, the government created the *Healthcare Safety Investigation Branch* of the *NHS Improvement* organisation, with the object of investigating matters of serious fraud. The government also created the *Health Service Safety Investigations Body (HSSIB)*, which has the task of investigating issues which specifically relate to patient safety.

The efficacy, objectivity, and independence of the HSSIB is yet to be proven but, if its effectiveness is anything like that of the Public Interest Disclosure Act, it will be little more than more propaganda, designed to make the public believe that the government are serious about acting in the public interest.

NHS Response to Whistleblowers

The NHS can follow two main strategies for "managing" whistleblowers, they can be proactive or reactive. Prior to being outlawed in 2019, the NHS could proactively prevent employees from whistleblowing by forcing them to sign non-disclosure agreements, known more commonly as "gagging orders". Since then, the only remaining proactive method is to employ or promote staff who will willingly comply with the cover-up culture of their employer. The reactive method, on the other hand, is to punish the whistleblower, either because they have blown the whistle, or to deter them from doing so. Punishment is never for whistleblowing, that would be illegal; instead, whistleblowers are punished for other reasons, which are most often of the "being aggressive towards colleagues" sort.

Punishing the whistleblower after they have blown the whistle seems like it is "closing the stable door after the horse has bolted", so seems to be a waste of time, but the punishment serves to discourage others from following the whistleblowing route, lest they also suffer career damaging revenge punishments, so it is a useful facility for management to deploy.

The superior method, for the NHS, is the proactive option of employing staff who will be willingly compliant with the institution's cover-up culture, and this is a popular and easy option. The type of people who support the cover-up culture are those who depend on the cover-up culture themselves and who are either not competent, are fraudulently qualified for their posts, or unsafe due to their drug or alcohol addictions.

As way of demonstration of positive career development and job security for unqualified staff, in return for devotion to the cover-up culture of their employer, the example of hospital T should prove insightful. Hospital T employs eight senior (band 7) anaesthetic technicians (ODPs). The official hospital specification of minimum **mandatory** educational attainment for band seven anaesthetic technicians and nurses is a Master's degree, yet not one of hospital T's band seven anaesthetic technicians is educated to a level above that of a primary school child of ten or eleven years old. Indeed, none of these senior employees has the ability to pass the British "Eleven-plus" test in English and mathematics, and none of them meet their Health and Care Professions Council registration requirement that they can calculate drug dosage problems – with a one hundred percent accuracy.

For the most senior anaesthetic technicians, of a major teaching hospital, to not have the basic numeracy skills that are meant to help ensure patient safety, is a such a corrupt and bizarre situation, that it easily deserves to be described by the popular expression of "you couldn't make it up!".

🚑 34: WHISTLEBLOWERS

Since 1998, the Public Interest Disclosure Act has been in place to encourage public sector workers to use the safety valve of whistleblowing to protect the public from matters related to safety and fraud, and to protect them from their employer's revenge punishments for doing so. The efficacy of the PID Act can be demonstrated by the effect, since then, the Act has had on whistleblowers – **no whistleblowers have been protected by the Public Interest Disclosure Act**.

The following short list illustrates the variety of experiences that public and NHS whistleblowers have suffered since the introduction of legal protection for making protected disclosures under the terms of the Public Interest Disclosure Act:

☿ Julie Bailey, "Cure The NHS"

Julie was a cafe owner who believed that NHS hospitals would act in the best interests of patients, and do whatever is necessary to improve their lives. After Julie's mother, Bella, was admitted to Staffordshire General Hospital, for a hiatus hernia, Julie learnt the truth about the attitude that the NHS has to individual patients – they are just numbers, whose hospital experience has to intersect with what is best for the image of NHS, and the meeting of targets for the hospital.

Bella Bailey's hospital admission proved to be a death sentence. Bella did not receive the basic standards of nursing care that meet the definition of nursing; she did not receive the oxygen therapy that she needed, she was not washed, watered, or fed; Bella's surgeon wanted to reduce his workload by allowing Bella to die, and asked her daughter, Julie, to sign a "Do not attempt resuscitation" form to allow that to happen. In one incident, Bella was lifted and carried by a healthcare assistant, a practice that is outlawed in the NHS, because it is considered dangerous for both patient and lifter", and proof of that is shown by the fact the healthcare assistant dropped Bella onto the floor and, as a consequent, Bella suffered damage to her heart. Inevitably, Bella's experience of "care" worsened her condition, and she died in hospital.

Julie then started her "Cure the NHS" campaign to draw attention to the public's attention to the true state of the NHS. Eventually, press coverage of Julie's campaign was too overwhelming for the government to ignore, so an inquiry was established. The inquiry concluded, amongst other things, that there was an absence of humanity, care, compassion, and no clinical or institutional leadership at Stafford General Hospital.

Doing what is best for patients is, usually, what helps protect the image of the NHS. However, doing what is best for an individual patient is not the hospital's primary goal but, rather, it is the meeting of government targets that has primacy and, by meeting those targets, the image of the government is protected.

8 Sharmila Chowdhury, Ealing Hospital

Sharmila was a Senior Radiographer, and Imaging Services Manager, for a department with sixty staff. One of her main duties was managing the department's budget, and ensuring that taxpayer's money was being properly spent.

When scrutinising the departmental accounts, Sharmila discovered a number of irregularities concerning some of the Radiologist Consultants. What she found was that a number of them had been persistently claiming fees for work they had not done, both from unworked overtime, and from claims that they worked on several days a week, when they were "moonlighting" at private hospitals.

Sharmila also discovered that the *Picture Archiving and Communication System* (PACS) manager had failed to upload six month's worth of clinical data, for a hundred or more patients. The potential consequences of out of date radiology information, for any of those critically ill patients, was extremely severe, and could easily have resulted in incorrect prognosis, treatment, and death.

After reporting her findings to senior management, as is the right and proper action, one of the fraudulent Consultants instructed the PACS Manager to make counter accusations against Sharmila, and she was dismissed, on the spot, and escorted out of the hospital.

Sharmila took legal action against the hospital which, in the vast majority of cases, is a pointless exercise, because the typical hospital response is to invoke the methods of the NHS cover-up culture, to deny wrongdoing, and "lose" evidence.

Prior to dismissal, Sharmila was smart enough to realise that she would become subject to management dirty tricks, so she ensured that she had possession of all of the documentary evidence that would substantiate her case. She won an Interim Relief Hearing, then an Appeal Hearing against Ealing Hospital, but the Chief Executive refused to reinstate her. Sharmila was then blacklisted, and found it unable to find work. Sharmila wrote an open letter to Jeremy Hunt (Health Secretary), and sent copies of the letter to a number of journalists. Jeremy Hunt used his influence to find her a job at Hammersmith Hospital, who put her in a role that she had no experience of, and which included doing the work of three people. Managers arranged things so that her life at Hammersmith would be as stressful and unpleasant as it could be, and she suffered both direct and indirect bullying. The stress of her experiences damaged Sharmila's immune system, and she developed cancer.

The crooked Consultants kept their jobs, were not investigated, and none of Sharmila's Imaging Department replacements have raised the issue of fraud – and their careers have thrived.

Details about Sharmila's case (well worth reading) are at:

-     **https://sharmilachowdhury.com**
-     **Twitter.com/sharmilaxx**

8 Dr Hayley Dare, West London Mental Health Trust

Violence and bullying against staff in the West London Mental Health Trust was reported as being the worst in the country. When psychologist Dr Dare raised this issue with management, and described how clinical staff were putting patients at risk through unsafe practices, managers started a malicious gossip campaign against her, with the aim of establishing a negative reputation about her professional competency, her mental health, and her poor social skills. Dr Dare also started receiving threatening letters, which advised her that there could be "consequences" to her children if she did not stop making disclosures. She did not back down, so she was dismissed from her job.

The Trust spent £120,000 of taxpayer's money on legal fees to defend their case, at an Employment Tribunal. Eventually, the law took the side of Dr Dare, and criticised the Trust for their hostility towards her, for acting in good faith, and their demands for £100,000 of legal costs, from Dr Dare, were dismissed.

8 Dr Chris Day, Queen Elizabeth Hospital

Chris, an intensive care doctor, reported to his superiors various patient safety concerns, particularly the raised risk to patients caused by understaffing. The response, by management and Health Education England, was to marshall the forces of the NHS to undermine and make false allegations against him.

Predictably, Dr Day's career has been badly, and permanently damaged by the NHS cover-up culture response to his attempts to improve patient safety. Indeed, it would be most unusual if that were not the case – such is the ruthlessness of the NHS.

Dr Day is in the process of legal action against the NHS, so it is too early to detail the full life cycle of his case but, so far, he has had some success in strengthening the law with regard to the rights of a junior doctor to raise patient safety issues.

8 Mr Peter Duffy, Royal Lancaster Infirmary

An award winning surgeon, who had saved the lives of many patients, blew the whistle, in 2015, on the incompetence of some fellow surgeons, who were brought to the UK on the strength of their claimed "qualifications" and surgical abilities. Some of the incidents, he reported to the Care Quality Commission, included ignoring emergency cases, because some other surgeons preferred to be paid for not working, and stay at home instead of being present at their designated places of work, with the result that some of those emergency cases resulted in unnecessary and avoidable death. Other examples of incompetence by Mr Duffy's three fellow surgeons included the intention to remove the wrong kidney for one patient, and a number of instances where these surgeons failed to diagnose cancer, and were unfamiliar with some basic tools of urology, such as ultrasound equipment.

The response to Mr Duffy's whistleblowing, by those he reported, was to claim that his motivations were based on racism against them (another old chestnut), which is an attempt to deflect from the matter that was raised. Managers then followed this up with the NHS standard bullying practice of gaslighting (psychological manipulation) and spreading malicious gossip about him, over a period of several years, culminating in his being forced out of his job. Even though Mr Duffy had the respect and affection of hospital staff, nobody would come forward to substantiate his case, such is the poisonous culture of the Royal Lancaster Infirmary. Mr Duffy was later awarded £102,000 compensation by an employment tribunal, and the claims of racism against him were deemed unfounded and unsubstantiated. More details of Mr Duffy's experiences have been reproduced in his book: *Whistle In The Wind*.

What is apposite about Mr Duffy's experience with foreign surgeons is the significant NHS "secret" of the Department of Health failing to properly screen them for proper qualifications and competencies. Many foreign doctors, of course, are as good as, or better than, their British counterparts, but it only takes a small fraction of the total number to ruin the lives of significant numbers of patients. Without effective screening for foreign doctors, of all types, before being let loose on patients, the patients become the "screeners" of the doctors who treat them, because the effectiveness of the treatment they receive is the test of efficacy. By then, of course, the damage is done and, if the "rogue" doctor can hide behind a protected title, as defined by the Equalities Act, then they will close down any complaints against them with claims of discrimination, and will only become disbarred after a series of poor patient outcomes, and associated trail of medical failures, makes their lack of competency too obvious to ignore.

8 Jennie Fecitt, Wythenshawe Walk-in Centre

Nurse Jennie Fecitt informed her bosses, in 2009, that one of her nurse colleagues had not been honest about his qualifications - he was treating adult patients, even though he was only qualified to work with children. Jennie was supported, in her complaint, by two other nurses, Annie Woodcock and Felicity Hughes.

After raising her concern, Jennie's daughter accepted a phone call, where she was told that her house would be burnt down, unless Jennie dropped her complaint. Jennie also experienced a campaign of malicious gossip against her which, in all likelihood, was meant to frighten her into acquiescence with management, or to "encourage" her to find alternative employment.

By now, readers will recognise the NHS pattern of behaviour here, in responding to staff concerns and disclosures, which can be summarised by: *Denial – Threaten – Intimidate - Smear campaign*. Clearly, the introduction of the Public Interest Disclosure Act, and promises of support from the government, towards whistleblowers, has had no effect on the hostile and cruel treatment that whistleblowers face.

Interestingly, to me at least, one of the early French phrases I learnt in my school days was "plus ça change, plus c'est la meme chose", which means "the more things change, the more things stay the same". I never understood the relevance of this phrase, until I started working in the NHS, because it describes, very well, how official expressions of intent to change things, and introducing laws and regulations to protect both patients and whistleblowers, are nothing more than political spin, designed to please the public when, in reality, nothing changes.

8 Sandra Haynes-Kirkbright

Sandra was head of Clinical Coding and Data Quality at New Cross Hospital, part of Royal Wolverhampton Trust, a role which requires ensuring the correct recording of the treatment types that patients receive, so that the hospital receives the proper funding for those treatments.

Shortly after taking up her post, Sandra discovered various coding discrepancies. Two major examples of which were the false classifying of "intracranial injury" for children who had precautionary overnight stays, and the changing of clinical codes for patients who, unexpectedly, died in hospital, to the state known as "palliative", which means they were officially classed as terminally ill patients who were only admitted for pain relief.

By classing children, who were kept overnight for precautionary observation, as suffering "intracranial injury", the hospital could claim more money from the government, than if the overnight stay was recorded for what it was – observation only.

For the patients who died, unexpectedly, classing them as "palliative" meant that the hospital's figure for their *Summary Hospital-level Mortality Indicator* was kept to a more "normal" level, and would help make it appear that the hospital's death rate not to be unusually high and, thereby, would not attract formal investigation or adverse publicity.

The Trust Chief Executive, Finance Director, and other senior figures failed to pressurise Sandra into complying with their fraud, and so they encouraged some of her colleagues to accuse her of bullying and abusive behaviour, giving management the excuse to suspend her, and make her seem unsuitable for employment elsewhere – she was blacklisted.

8 Marjan Jahangiri, St George's Hospital Trust

In 2017, the National Institute for Cardiovascular Outcomes Research (NICOR) alerted St George's of the high death rate of patients at the cardiac (heart surgery) unit, which were more than double the national average. In 2018, Professor Jahangiri, one of the hospitals's heart surgeons, was suspended from her post, for shouting at a nurse. Professor Jahangiri took legal action against the Trust, and won her case at a High Court Hearing. At that Hearing, Mr Justice Nicklin criticised the St George's Trust for taking disciplinary action against Professor Jahangiri, based on evidence (from the nurse) that the Medical Director, Professor Andrew Rhodes, did not receive until two weeks after her suspension. Additionally, Justice Nicklin criticised the Chief Executive, Jacqueline Totterdell, for deciding to take annual leave whilst the disciplinary case was ongoing, even though she had ultimate responsibility in making decisions about suspension and exclusion of Consultants, such as Professor Jahangiri.

⚲   ⚲   ⚲

During this time, there was a lot of rivalry and aggression between surgeons in the cardiac unit, and there were also complaints that some surgeons were cancelling NHS patients, in favour of more lucrative private cases. Together with the NICOR alert of high deaths, these factors threatened to immerse St George's in a lot of bad publicity and, so, to protect themselves, senior management appeared to use Professor Jahangiri as a scapegoat for the NICOR report, and the consequential shutting down of the cardiac unit.

Notably, Justice Nicklin's criticised Jacqueline Totterdell's (Chief Executive) attempts to absolve herself of being involved in the case against Professor Jahangiri, can be also applied to her role in the Covid-19 pandemic, where she decided to pass on her duties to an assistant, whilst she self isolated, at home, between March and September, 2020. To make it appear that she was justified in keeping away from work, Totterdell spread the rumour that she had a health problem that made her vulnerable to Covid-19, and substantiated it by using the fact that she had an operation in November 2019. That operation was of a cosmetic nature, and she could have returned to work a week later, but she took sick leave until the start of the official lockdown – a period of four months, giving a total of ten months off work, and on full pay.

❡ ❡ ❡

During her Court case, Professor Jahangiri told Mr Justice Nicklin that the hospital was more interested in enforcing their cover-up culture than focusing on patient care. She also revealed that St George's, who were represented by their Reputation Manangement lawyers (Capsticks Law) had a culture of bullying staff who spoke out about safety and care issues and, in an attempt to frighten her into silence, she was sent a dead rat and a decapitated doll in the post.

Following Justice Nicklin's ruling in Professor Jahangiri's favour, and criticisms of St George's Medical Director and Chief Executive, the Medical Director lost his Directorship, and is now working as an anaesthetist at St George's. The Chief Executive is still in post.

❡ ❡ ❡

This case illustrates the way St George's management and Directors deal with the most important issue, which is patient safety and, specifically, the problem of high cardiac patient mortality, by looking for scapegoats to deflect from, and blame for, the dysfunctional and toxic atmosphere which permeates all parts of the hospital, rather than focussing their efforts on resolving the clinical and inter-personal causes of the high patient mortality.

In the intervening sixteen years between this and the Ian Parkin case (next), the cover-up and bullying culture of St George's Hospital does not appear to have changed, and no government bodies have done anything to correct this situation.

8 Ian Parkin, St George's Hospital (Tooting)

Ian Parkin had been the hospital's Finance Director for twelve years, prior to his dismissal in 2002, for being aggressive and having a poor management style. Ian's dismissal came after he reported to his Board of Directors that his junior staff had been forced into changing weekly reports to show that no surgical operations had been cancelled when, in fact, there were sometimes as many as thirty cancellations a week. Ian's case was raised in Prime Minister's Question Time, but no government official wanted to address the problem of figures being fiddled, perhaps because it was the government that benefitted from those false figures.

8 Gary Walker, Lincoln County Hospital

In 2009, when he was the Chief Executive of Lincoln County Hospital, Gary Walker reported to the East Midlands Health Authority the problem of not being able to meet the government target of treating patients within the specified eighteen weeks - his hospital did not have the capacity to meet demand. He was threatened that, if he did not provide reports that showed that Lincoln Hospital was meeting its targets, the Strategic Health Authority would cancel a planned extra eleven million pounds of funding for his hospital.

Gary Walker refused to either fiddle the figures, which would be fraudulent, or to rush patients through the system, because that would be dangerous for the patients. In 2010, Gary was dismissed from his post, officially, for swearing and being aggressive towards his colleagues. To preserve the image of the Health Authority, Gary was made to "keep quiet" by signing a non-disclosure agreement.

One year prior to Gary Walker's dismissal, the Lincoln County Hospital Chairman, David Bowles, quit his post because he was also pressured into ensuring that published targets met government expectations. He described the NHS as having a bullying and cruel culture, and highlighted the types of pressure he faced, including personal threats to him and his family.

APPENDICES

ᐭ Appendix 1: NHS Cover-up Methods

For a patient, who has been subject to a poor medical outcome, resulting from treatment in the NHS, understanding how the truth about their treatment may have been hidden from them can make the difference between them winning and losing a case of culpability, so being familiar with the machinations of the NHS cover-up culture is fundamental to defending against it.

To understand how the truth about a particular medical case has been concealed or disguised, it is necessary to be familiar with certain aspects of the cover-up culture; specifically:

(a) What the cover-up culture is.

(b) How the cover-up culture works.

(c) Who benefits from cover-ups.

(d) Who suffers from cover-ups.

(a) The cover-up culture is the endemic NHS response to hiding the truth about any issue that would reflect badly on the various NHS managers and officials in the NHS hierarchy, all the way up to the higher echelons of government. Hiding the truth about an issue can take the form of concealment, diversion, disguise, deflection, denial, and broadcasting false information.

(b) The cover-up culture is composed of a triad of factors:

(i) The techniques of deception which, as previously mentioned, are grouped under the umbrella term of "**Maskirovka**".

(ii) The practice of feeding the public with false or misleading information, using the methods of **propaganda**.

(iii) **Bullying**, which has the aim of deterring staff from revealing the truth about the above deception and propaganda.

(c) The NHS cover-up culture protects and benefits the people who are responsible for delivering the service that patients receive. Quite simply, if service delivery is sub-standard, the officials holding the responsibility for that service are at risk of losing their positions and status, so, burying bad news helps maintain their job security.

(d) The targets who suffer from the cover-up culture are the service consumers – the patients, and the people who deliver the service - the staff. When the quality and effects of a patient's medical experience have proven to be less than what could be reasonably expected, the covering up of the truth of that case might mean that the patient, or their estate, will not be eligible for proper compensation and, for clinical staff, hiding the issue can result in a missed opportunity to learn lessons from the case.

📖 📖 📖 📖 📖

When considering any NHS issue that may have involved a cover-up, a greater understanding of the problem might be gained by decomposing the issue into the three factors that constitute the cover-up process, repeated and emphasised here:

NHS Triad of Cover-up Factors

Maskirovka – deception or concealment of truth.

Propaganda – replace negative true news with positive false news, commonly referred to as "spin".

Bullying – protects and preserves propaganda and maskirovka.

Understanding the above three components of a covered-up issue can help the investigator, either the patient or the patient's advocate, to strengthen the case they may have against their antagonist which, typically, will be a particular hospital.

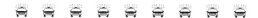

ᕲ Appendix 2: Maskirovka Explained

The NHS is characterised by its cover-up culture, but the term "cover-up" does not accurately describe how, or the extent to which, issues are effectively hidden from the public. "Covering up" suggests the concealment of something, but NHS officials cannot completely conceal everything they want to hide. In most cases, officials have to employ secondary techniques that are better described by the philosophy and techniques of *maskirovka.*

Maskirovka is the Russian word for "masking", and is the process of concealing assets, behaviours, events, and intentions. Maskirovka's relevance to the NHS is significant, because it matches the suite of methods that the NHS uses to conceal the truth about its culture, and the poor care that some patients receive.

Concealing an issue is the gold standard for implementing the maskirovka aspect of the NHS cover-up culture but, when it is not possible to completely hide a particular issue, then secondary techniques of maskirovka are used to conceal what is the target of the "cover up", with the principle secondary techniques being diversion, disguise, and deflection.

Applied Maskirovka

Targets: Assets, Behaviours, Events, Intentions.

Aims: Conceal, Divert, Disguise, Deflect.

Methods: Denial, Propaganda, Dead Cat Strategy, Gaslighting.

To achieve their **aim**, the maskirovka executor will apply one or more of the above **methods**, as explained next:

🕸 Aims of **Maskirovka**

⚓ **Concealing** an issue is the ideal, but most difficult, aim of the maskirovka executor – if nobody knows about it, investigations will never occur. A popular method to conceal an issue is denial.

⚓ **Diversion** is misdirection by focusing attention way from the issue being covered up, and towards another matter (dead cat on the table), such as what happens when politicians "bury bad news" by drawing attention to some other more sensational issue.

⚓ **Disguising** issues that reflect badly on the NHS or government is a common practice and occurs when, for example, a medical mistake resulting in a patient death is disguised by false information, recording it as "age related", or the patient's admission is officially classed as "palliative".

⚓ **Deflection** from the issue is what can happen to an employee who raises an issue of concern – management will assign blame elsewhere, or make false accusations, against the employee, of incompetence, or bullying, and use propaganda (malicious gossip campaign) against them. Alternatively, the employee can be "gaslighted". Subsequently, the employee is too occupied with their own professional survival and wellbeing to devote effort to the matter that they originally raised.

Methods of Maskirovka

Denial is the most easy to understand method of maskirovka, because it is used so frequently. For example, if someone retrospectively tabulates a patient's clinical record with fake values, and there is no definitive proof of what they did, the perpetrator will deny what they have done. In an instance of bullying, the bully will deny their behaviour and, in many instances, try to reverse the bully/victim roles, using the principle of DARVO (*refer to the chapter on BULLYING & HARASSMENT*).

Propaganda can be used to meet any of the aims (Conceal, Divert, Disguise, Deflect) of the executor. The NHS produces a constant stream of propaganda, using all forms of media – newspapers, public announcements, government statistics for clinical targets, and social media. *Freedom To Speak Up Guardians*, for example, are prolific with their announcements about how effective they are in protecting whistleblowers. (Another popular propaganda technique is illustrated in Appendix 4)

Dead Cat Strategy means deflecting from one issue to another issue that is more shocking or interesting. For example, when a hospital is publically outed for high death rates, the NHS may claim that critics have a history of corruption and political agitation and are, therefore, acting against the public interest.

🜨 Gaslighting is also a commonly used technique, and is what a manipulator does to make their victim doubt what they know is true, and even doubt their sanity, by diverting their attention onto their own failures and psychological weaknesses. When NHS managers "encourage" a whistleblower's colleagues to socially exclude them, it has the intention of making the victim believe that there is something wrong with their behaviours, situational and event awareness, and social skills.

Gaslighting can also be achieved through persistent denial – if enough people tell a lie often enough, it can become "fact" to their victim. Another commonly used diversionary tactic against NHS targets of management ire, is to sabotage the work they do by, for example, removing or incapacitating equipment that they have previously checked as being functional and appropriate.

🜨 Maskirovka and the NHS

The philosphy of cover-ups, using the techniques of maskirovka, is part of the virtual ethos of the NHS, and is the natural way that the organisation deals with information that may reflect NHS officials, and the government, in a bad light.

Describing the NHS as having a cover-up culture, incidentally, is not a subjective derogatory description, it is a term that was formally recognised by a former Health Secretary, Jeremy Hunt, after publication of a 2014 damning report by Lord Francis:

"1,000 patients a month are dying needlessly in NHS hospitals

because of staff blunders." the Health Secretary has warned, as he announces "sweeping reforms to bring an end to a 'cover-up culture' which is risking lives." Jeremy Hunt, 2015.

⚜ Appendix 3: Propaganda Techniques

The primary theme of this book is the cover-up culture of the NHS, where true information of public interest is concealed or manipulated. Suppressing truth about the NHS, ultimately, protects the public image of the government and NHS, and helps secure the careers of those who conceal such information.

The widespread practice of concealing the truth about the NHS was acknowledged at the Global Patient Safety Summit (March 2016), when the Health Secretary, Jeremy Hunt, announced the government's intention to end the NHS cover-up culture, and to provide protection from disciplinary action against employees who raise concerns. Predictably, nothing meaningful has developed to tackle this cover-up culture; Jeremy Hunt's expressions may simply be a case of government "spin". However, by acknowledging that the NHS cover-up culture exists, it is no longer possible for NHS officials to ignore the matter, or to deny its existence. It is, at least, a first step.

* * *

In recent world history, tools of deception have often included the techniques of propaganda - dovetails neatly with maskirovka - and the value of propaganda can be best illustrated by its use in Nazi Germany. Adolf Hitler sang the praises of propaganda in his book, *Mein Kampf*, where he expressed his belief that propaganda was essential in influencing and controlling the population. Prior to Hitler becoming Chancellor, he appointed Joseph Goebbels to be the controller of all Nazi Party information, and the architect of all misinformation campaigns, with the aim of supporting Hitler's political and military ambitions. The Nazi propaganda machine was so notably effective, that the messages it espoused are still believed by some, to this day. Although Hitler was defeated, militarily, his successful use of propaganda has become a "normal" part of military, political, and business life, albeit disguised as, for example, public relations, "spin", or advertising artistic license. Indeed, propaganda, by any other name, is the primary weapon in the arsenal of any government's strategy of convincing the electorate to vote for them.

In the United Kingdom, one of the most significant general election vote winning factors is healthcare provision by the NHS, and all political parties have to convince the public that they are keen defenders of the NHS, if they are to attract their votes. To do this, governments rely heavily on propaganda, both *black* and *white.*

White propaganda means making a persuasive claim with the support of selected facts which are generally accepted as being valid. Alternatively, *black* propaganda is based on fake or unprovable "facts". *Gray* propaganda is used to describe propaganda that is not so easily classified as either black or white.

To better understand how the NHS uses propaganda, it is useful to understand some general propaganda methods, and how they complement or repeat the practice of maskirovka. For illustration purposes, assume you, the reader, are the propagandist.

⊛ Methods of the Propagandist

⊕ 1. Learn the beliefs of the target.

If you (the propagandist) do not understand your target, you will not be able to manipulate their thinking. Learn their beliefs, but do not let the target know that you are aware of their beliefs; it is better to let the target reveal that their beliefs match yours.

⊕ 2. Hook the target.

Use sensationalism to get the target's attention. If the target believes that "fact" X is false, make the claim that your opponent believes that fact "X" is true. Better still, make the assertion that your opponent condemns anyone who believes that X is false, thereby reinforcing this rule with rule 5.

⊕ 3. Get the target to agree with their own beliefs.

By asking the target to agree with things which you already know they agree with, they will be more inclined to agree with other matters which you present to them (rule 4).

⊕ 4. Claim the same beliefs as the target.

If you know (surreptitiously) that the target believes that issue A is true, announce that you believe that A is true, thereby making the target think you are more likely to act in their interests, because you have the same beliefs.

⊕ 5. Appeal to the target's emotions.

To draw the target into your belief system, use their emotions to let them conclude what you want them to conclude, rather than use facts to persuade them to your way of thinking. Example emotions are fear, safety, hatred, and greed.

✪ 6. Never disagree with the target.

If you are not in complete agreement with the target, they might assume that your belief systems are not compatible. Additionally, disagreement means method 4 is compromised.

✪ 7. Be selective with information.

Do not reveal all relevant information, if it paints an accurate picture of the matter at hand – be selective with what you present. This is probably the most frequently used tactic in politics and advertising, and is easily demonstrated with food product sales campaigns, such as: Food product A has a new label which states "Now with 25% less fat!". In this example, the previous product A recipe contained 800 calories, and the new recipe has only 600 calories, making it more appealing than product B, which has not been reduced in calories. The manufacturer has been truthful in their calorie reduction claim for product A, but they do not reveal that product B only has 500 calories, making it (still) less fattening than product A.

This rule is used against NHS employees in disciplinary processes, and is realised by using snippets of information in contexts that harm the accused employee, whilst simultaneously disallowing information that negates those negative snippets. Psychologists refer to this behaviour as "confirmation bias".

✪ 8. If propaganda "facts" cannot be validated, do not reveal the source of those "facts".

This is a simple tactic of using lies and gossip to support a claim, or to undermine an opponent.

✸ 9. Reveal credible sources of information.

This is *white* propaganda, which can be as basic as quoting a publicly made statement by an official spokesman, or providing documentary evidence from an apparently reputable source to support a claim. An example of this rule is where a salesman informs a crowd of shoppers that he is selling a particular perfume, which is advertised for sale in a popular women's magazine (credible source), with an advertised sale price of £200, for the knock down price of only £8. The fact that this same perfume is advertised in a well known publication makes it seem a bargain buy. What the shoppers don't know is that the perfume is just water and diluted cheap perfume, bought by the container load, at a cost of £1 a bottle, and the advertisment was placed by the salesman, to make it appear to be an expensive product. An analogy with the NHS is that of behind the scenes television programmes, that show the positive and human side of the health service, and evoke predictable responses (compassion and respect) in the audience. It's on TV, so it must be genuine! With respect to the common issue of punishing staff who raise concerns, malicious gossip about the staff member, to destroy their credibility, is substantiated by claims that that there are credible witnesses to that person's aggression, incompetence etc, so it must be true?

✸ 10. Evoke predictable responses in the target.

If the aim of a propaganda campaign is to manipulate the feelings of a target towards a particular emotion, then feed them information which stimulates that emotion. So, if you want the target to feel that politician "A" is kind and caring, and politician "B" is cruel and uncaring, let the target believe that politician "A" intends to allocate resources to children suffering from condition "X" (also suffered by the target's child), but politician "B" has no such intent. The target's predictable response will be disgust and hatred for politician "B".

✸ 11. Emphasise the object of aggression.

This is where a propaganda campaign has the aim of discrediting an opponent – the object of aggression – by linking them to negative issues and events. An example of this type is that of the personal attacks made by the EU "remain" supporters, on Boris Johnson, during the so called "Brexit" process. The "remainers" do not want to alienate the voters who support Brexit, who are in the majority, and any criticism of them will mean a loss of votes for those parties who have attacked the Brexit voters. Instead, they focus on the personality and private life of Boris Johnson, because those issues are independent of politics. (This is another "dead cat" strategy.)

✸ 12. Create a simple mantra.

Convey your message in a manner that does not require explanation, and is easy to remember. To continue the Brexit example, the mantra of the "remain" camp - "Crash out of the EU" - was intended to appeal to the emotions of voters by using "crash" to associate leaving the EU with the pain and injury of a car crash. The Brexit supporting politicians also used propaganda of emotion to appeal to voters, with the mantra "Get Brexit done", because they knew that voters were frustrated and annoyed with the way the Brexit process was being delayed and sabotaged, so much so that the British parliamentary process became an international embarrassment. Both camps used mantras to appeal to voters – both sides used propaganda.

✸ 13. Facts by repetition.

If enough people make a false statement often enough, what they claim will eventually assume the status of being a "fact". The practice of "gaslighting" uses this rule.

14. Criticise opponent repeatedly.

This rule uses rule 13 to discredit an opponent.

15. Link beliefs with heroes.

Associate your beliefs with those of someone, such as a celebrity or scientist, who the target respects or trusts. Similarly, illustrate how someone who your target does not like or respect is associated with a position which is contrary to yours.

16. Join the crowd.

If the target is the type of person who wants to fit in and be accepted as being part of the "crowd", rather then being seen as an outsider, make them think that you (the propagandist) are part of that crowd, and your beliefs are the majority beliefs.

17. Divert and Deflect attention.

To deter a target from focussing on something which is sensitive to you, shift attention to some other issue, and publish information which gives the other issue credibility. This technique is the Maskirovka "dead cat strategy", which means diverting from an issue by introducing a distraction. The "dead cat strategy" is used by NHS managers when an employee raises an issue which managers prefers to be hidden - managers deflect from the issue by making false accusations against the employee. Officials will also deflect attention away from a patient or staff member's complaint, by claiming they are unbalanced, or have mental health issues. Doctors, managers,

PALS - will say anything to shift the focus from the issue raised.

⬡ 18. Fail to keep a promise – pass the blame.

Draw in the target's support by making a false promise of action that benefits them, then use the excuse that an opponent has sabotaged the action, or make the claim that a change of circumstances have made the promise inactionable (*Example: Government promises "we won't raise taxes", then renege because world events have changed*).

When a politician or NHS official makes a statement regarding, for example, policy or delivery of service by the NHS or other public body, the statement will use some of the above propaganda rules to support their arguments and claims that they are acting in the best interests of service users. Most notably, these rules are executed in election campaigns where the object of the propagandist is to convince the public that the NHS is safest in their hands, but is at risk if left under the control of any of the opposition parties.

Similarly, when an NHS employee or member of the public makes a complaint about the NHS, either to a body such as the CQC, or to the NHS itself, the response will also contain elements of the above rules of propaganda (particularly 1, 4, 5, 7, 8, 10, 17) which, in general, has the aim of closing down the complaint and, as long as rule 6 is not compromised, will often be successful.

The complainant, subject to the propaganda, must recognise these rules, if they are to continue their complaint without wrongly being convinced that their concerns are being properly addressed.

ᨆ Appendix 4: Television Propaganda

Governments use the NHS as vehicle for propaganda, by allowing hospitals to give television access to the clinical experiences of patients. The producers of these programmes have the object of attracting as many viewers as they can, and they do so by drawing viewers into feeling empathy with the televised patients and their families. This empathy is triggered when the viewing families watch how the families featured on the television show suffer the shock and fear that occurs when a family member is taken dangerously ill, and then receives life-saving medical intervention which, ultimately, leads to a positive return to health for that family member.

ᨏ Implementation of Propaganda Rules

ᨐ Rule 2: Hook the target.

Draw the public's attention by showing a dangerously ill trauma patient whose survival is entrusted to the NHS.

ᨐ Rule 4: Claim the same beliefs as the target.

The government know that the public believe that the NHS should be maintained, so the government strategy is to make the public think that the they also believe that the NHS is worth preserving.

❀ Rule 5: Appeal to the target's emotions.

Make the audience feel empathy with the plight of the patient and their family, by letting them see the family upset and fearful that their loved one might die. Viewers will automatically imagine themselves in the same situation, and will associate the experiences of the featured family with what could happen to them.

❀ Rule 7: Be selective with information.

Do not show any clinical failures or other negative issues, such as avoidable mistakes, staff shortages, poor services, low staff morale, or any other matter that the NHS and government officials would prefer to remain concealed from the public.

❀ Rule 10: Evoke predictable responses.

The patient's successful life saving treatment will be demonstrated, along with subsequent resumption of a normal and happy life for all the family. The family's gratitude to the NHS, and trust in the government to continue to maintain NHS efficacy, will be propagated to the viewing audience.

❀ Rule 13: Create facts by repetition.

The recurring broadcasting of such television programmes has the overt intention of reinforcing the public's confidence in the NHS, and the covert intention to convince the public that it is the government who make the NHS such an effective body, and whose commitment to the NHS is assured.

The overall aim of the above propaganda scheme is to fix, in the minds of the public, the "fact" that, regardless of whatever else the government has done, or failed to do, at least the NHS is safe in their hands, and that might be enough to convince enough floating voters, at the time of the general election, to swing the votes in the direction of the government.

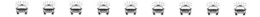

ᘓ Appendix 5: Precautionary Principle

One of the defining historical attitudes towards safety, of the British government and its arms, is that everything is classed as "safe" by default, and that the safe status of any object or circumstance does not change, until definitive evidence proves otherwise. The proof of something not being safe usually comes into existence when someone suffers significant harm, caused by the particular object or circumstance which, too frequently, means someone has to die before the matter is accepted as being not safe, and before mitigating action is taken to prevent a recurrence of the same unsafe situation.

This is the pattern of behaviour towards safety that is adopted by the NHS: don't take the necessary precautions to prevent a death or other mishap, unless those precautions are either mandated or conform to minimum codes of practice or, if by failing to take precautions, they will adversely affect "targets". An easy way to illustrate the failure to behave in a precautionary manner is to use the example of the well publicised event, where nearly two hundred people died - the *Herald of Free Enterprise* disaster.

It may seem incongruous to discuss a maritime disaster in a book about the NHS but, after reading this account, the reader will have the *Precautionary Principle* firmly ingrained in their minds, and will better appreciate why so many NHS blunders could have so easily been avoided, if only this simple principle was followed.

📇 Cross Channel Ferry Dangers

When a roll-on/roll-off ferry loads and unloads its cargo of passengers and vehicles, the time spent, in harbour, does not generate revenue, and the costs incurred when using jetty space is determined by time spent alongside. There is, consequently, a financial imperative to minimise the time spent moored up to a jetty. One way to reduce the amount of time being moored up is to set sail before it is properly safe to do so which, in this specific example, means setting sail before the vehicle decks have been cleared of toxic and inflammable exhaust fumes; ferries would set sail with both bow and stern vehicle deck doors (only a few feet above the water line) open, so that the breeze would flush out the vehicle exhaust fumes.

If the ferry was perfectly ballasted, the sea conditions were perfectly flat, and there was no wind, the ferry could set sail without incident. Alternatively, if less than perfect conditions existed, there was the chance that even a slight swell (wave height) could cause water ingress into the vehicle deck and, with just a few inches of water, the stability of the ferry could cause it to capsize. This possibility was repeatedly reported to the Department of Transport and the ferry owners, over a number of years, by passengers and mariners alike, but the practice was not made illegal, or defined as bad practice, and so it continued to be "allowed". In March, 1987, this situation changed.

🚗 Herald of Free Enterprise

The roll-on/roll-off car ferry, *Herald of Free Enterprise*, slipped her moorings in the port of Zeebrugge, Belgium, and set sail for Dover. Both its bow and stern vehicle deck doors were left open, to exhaust the toxic vehicle fumes from the vehicle deck. Before the ship reached as far as Zeebrugge harbour entrance, the bow dipped under water and scooped up enough water to capsize the vessel, and one hundred and ninety-three passengers, including a number of babies and children, drowned.

After this event, the practice of sailing with hull doors open was outlawed. The change in the law was a typical reactive step, and is in line with the above mentioned British practice of waiting for someone to die before something is classified as being not safe.

🚗 Precautionary Principle & Safety

Since 1991, UK Health and Safety legislation has been complemented by the **Precautionary Principle**, which is meant to prevent recurrence of Zeebrugge ferry type disasters.

> "The purpose of the Precautionary Principle is to create an impetus to take a decision not withstanding scientific uncertainty about the nature and extent of the risk, i.e. to avoid 'paralysis by analysis' by removing excuses for inaction on the grounds of scientific uncertainty." **Health and Safety Executive, 2018.**

What the Precautionary Principle means, in simple terms, is that instead of requiring that the person who voices their concern to the body (ferry operator and government) who holds the risk, having to provide proof that a hazard and its associated risk exists, the burdon of proof lies with the risk holder to prove that the hazard does **not** exist, or that its associated risk is as low as is reasonably practicable. This can be simplified even further by saying *the body creating the risk is guilty of safety violations by default.*

❧ Precautionary Principle and the NHS

In the NHS, the Precautionary Principle, in the main, is neither complied with, or known by managers, team leaders, hospital directors, or NHS officials. This is one of the reasons that employees, who "blow the whistle", are met with management assertions that the particular hazard does not exist, using the fact that there is no history of the particular issue causing harm. Managers will only take mitigating actions after the hazard has been realised, and someone has suffered harm, or a reportable "never event" has occurred.

It might be difficult to understand why a manager would tolerate potentially unsafe situations, but, acknowledging a problem means managing the problem, and that would mean reporting the issue to a more senior level of management which, in turn, means partially or wholly transferring responsibility up the chain of command. In the NHS, protecting more senior staff from issues, which they would prefer not to know about, is an unwritten part of the duty of a person who is immediately subordinate to that more senior person.

All levels of management want the comfort and security of a "hear no evil, see no evil" environment – if they don't know about the issue, they will not be found culpable if harm comes to a patient. If a senior person does know, officially, about a safety issue, and they do not do anything about it, then realisation of the particular dangerous event means that they will have to justify their lack of mitigating actions that would have prevented the risk event from occurring. The senior person will not be able to pass the blame onto a subordinate, and their job might be at risk, and that is the underlying objective of a manager – to protect their job.

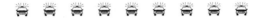

6⁄ Appendix 6: Equalities Act

I n the United Kingdom, equality legislation is served by the Equalities Act (2010), with the express purpose of ensuring and promoting a fair and equal society, and to provide legal protection from discrimination for anyone who possesses particular characteristics, such as gender, age, etc., known as *Protected Titles*. This legislation should ensure that no worker suffers disadvantage because they do not have equality with their colleagues.

In the NHS, managers and personnel department clerks are very selective with how they comply with the Equalities Act, and employees do not have any real protection from discrimination or any other type of unequal treatment. If anyone genuinely feels that they are not being treated according to the terms and spirit of the Equalities Act, and they attempt to address the issue, by following a complaints procedure, they will be seen as posing a threat to the NHS cover-up culture. Managers and directors prefer not to employ people who have the temerity to stand up for themselves, primarily because those are the type of people who are more likely to also stand up for patients, and that might mean speaking out about matters that management would prefer to keep from the public, particularly in regard to patient deaths and other poor outcomes.

Protected Titles

Age
Disability
Gender reassignment
Race
Religion
Sex
Sexual orientation

🚑 Minimal Compliance

In the NHS, the Equalities Act is complied with on the basis of minimality, which means only when it cannot be avoided, and then, only to meet the letter of the law – not the spirit.

Evidence of this can be seen with recruitment and promotion practices, where managers smoothe the career paths for those they favour, either for personal, professional, or discriminatory reasons, and lip service is paid to the requirements of the Equalites Act. Ignoring the requirements of equality legislation is not difficult, especially as the act, itself, has a number of flaws; described next.

💣 Equality Act Failures

🚑 Equality Failure 1

The Equalities Act does not prevent discrimination, and does not incorporate any facility for detection of discrimination. If someone is discriminated against, that individual must take legal action to prove discrimination against them, and that means spending a great deal of money on legal representation which, if unsuccessful, can bankrupt the person making the claim of discrimination. That is why publicity regarding successful discrimination claims is mostly limited to wealthy and well connected people. It is rare for a working class person to have any such success.

Equality Failure 2

The Equalities Act is not a deterrence to discrimination against someone having a protected title, especially in the NHS, because being found guilty of contravening the Equalities Act does not impose a custodial sentence or financial penalty on any manager or director who is guilty of the discrimination. Instead, if the NHS employer (hospital) is found guilty of contravening the Equalities Act - which rarely happens – the employer would have to pay any financial penalty, which means it is the taxpayer who pays the fine.

Equality Failure 3

If someone makes a claim of discrimination, whether they win or lose, a gossip campaign against them will make them become unemployable, because that person will be considered too much of a strong character to intimidate into keeping quiet about how their employer treats them or their colleagues, in terms of discrimination, or any other matter. Notably, this would not be the situation for a hospital which complies with the letter and spirit of equality legislation, but no NHS employee would expect any part of the NHS to make such compliance, so the risk of being "black-listed" is known by all employees, and that is a significant deterrence to making a claim of discrimination.

🚐 Equality Failure 4

The Equalities Act fails in one respect more than any other. Specifically, by making it illegal to discriminate only on the grounds of the stated *Protected Titles*, other types of discrimination are allowed – by law. A hospital can, for instance, deny employment to one person for being a fan of a particular football team, having a hairstyle which the manager is jealous of (this has happened), or for being better educated than the manager (take note - Pilgrm Hospital Operating Theatre Dept). Fans of the "Family Guy" cartoon may be familiar with an episode where the perfect female candidate for a job was unsuccessful, because the male interviewer preferred to select the female candidate with the "best chest". That may only be a cartoon story but, under British anti-discrimination legislation, it is perfectly legal to discriminate on that basis.

🚐 Equality Failure 5

The Equalities Act fails to address another aspect of discrimination, and that is the issue of favouritism. As already discussed, NHS favouritism, which is discrimination by indirect means, is just as prevalent as discrimination, and is something which continues, because it is not illegal to do so. Unlike direct discrimination, which is felt and detected by the victim, favouritism only becomes obvious by looking at the demographics of the people who are employed in a particular workplace. One very obvious example of favouritism occurs at the Operating Theatre Department of hospital T, where there is a disproportionate number of senior clinical staff who are young, blonde, and female. Conversely, there is a disproportionately high fraction of band five (lowest band) clinical staff, who are much more experienced and capable than the young blondes, but have no possibility of promotion or other career development opportunities, because those opportunities are reserved for the "blondes". Perhaps a politician, who might be genuinely concerned about the lack of equality in the NHS, specifically, or in British society, generally, might consider proposing a new law: the **Anti-Favouritism Act**.

♻ Appendix 7: Natural Justice

According to the UK Parliament's *Independent Complaints and Grievance Policy Proposals*, "The principles of natural justice concern procedural fairness and ensure a fair decision is reached by an objective decision maker. Maintaining procedural fairness protects the rights of individuals and enhances public confidence in the process."

Natural Justice principles consist of three rules, all of which must be applied, if the object (employee) of disciplinary action is to suffer investigations or disciplinary actions:

♣ The Hearing Rule

This is the requirement that the defendant (the accused) has the opportunity to present their case against the plaintiff (the accuser).

♣ The Bias Rule

Neither the accuser, or anyone who has a mutual interest with the accuser, must be involved with the decision making and judgements in the case. If a manager (accuser) makes an accusation against an employee (accused), the manager must not have any influence in the judgement, and the person making the judgement must not have any bias in favour of the manager.

♠ The Evidence Rule

Judgements must be based on tangible evidence and proof, and not on speculation. Additionally, evidence, in all of its forms, must be available for scrutiny by both parties. If evidence, real or fabricated, is used against the defendant, without the defendant having access to that evidence, the Evidence rule is compromised, and action against the defendant must be withdrawn.

♣ NHS Staff

The principles of natural justice are not considered in NHS disciplinary cases, and employees are never informed of these basic rights; the authority and power of managers and personnel departments is corrupt and autocratic, and is meant to impose the will of management, rather than determine the truth of accusations made against employees. Potential whistleblowers, especially, should be aware of their rights to natural justice, because, when they suffer the inevitable disciplinary action for their whistleblowing - dressed as some other matter - they can use the absence of natural justice principles, in their disciplinary cases, as a weapon with which to counter-attack their employer, at any independent and valid employment tribunal. This is an important issue, because NHS employers are afraid of laundering their dirty washing in public, that is why they punish whistleblowers – to frighten them into acquiescence with the cover-up culture.

An understanding of natural justice, therefore, should be the linchpin for a disciplined employee's attack on the unfair disciplinary process that they are subjected to because, in the NHS, attack is the only form of defence that an employee has a chance of being effective.

ᕲᒧ Appendix 8: Increased Risk Factors

S ome of the main factors that increase risk to patients in surgical and maternity care include:

♿ Shortage of staff: Surgeons, Anaesthetists, Midwives, Nurses, Operating Department Practitioners (ODPs).

♿ Low ratio of experienced to inexperienced staff.

♿ Minimal or no support for junior staff.

♿ Bullying and blame culture dissuade staff from admitting mistakes, or asking for assistance.

♿ Low standards of education and intelligence for nurses, midwives, and ODPs, resulting in staff (with exceptions) with limited ability to analyse and understand the patient condition. *This problem will not be resolved unless more capable people are attracted to these careers, and that cannot happen without a significant increase in pay, conditions, equality, and prospects.*

♿ Reluctance of doctors to discuss and share information with other staff (midwives etc), due to lack of respect, and the "class" distinction between doctors and other staff.

♿ Staff unable to understand regulations, paperwork, due to dyslexia or lack of English ability.

♿ Some foreign doctors do not treat patients as equals, and will not tolerate questioning by patients. *This is a failure of the NHS to ensure all staff understand British principles of equality, fairness, and respect.*

♿ Targets that put pressure on staff to rush patients through the system – quantity over quality.

♿ Inadequate Informed Consent, and clinical options not explained sufficiently, or accurately recorded.

♿ Reduced ability of staff due to fatigue, caused by long shifts and irregular shift patterns.

♿ Staff unable to focus on patient care due to being distracted by stress of bullying, favouritism, and pressure to cover-up incidents.

♿ No possibility of honest and impartial second opinions for clinical conditions and courses of treatment.

♿ Shortage of Ward Beds.

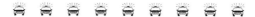

ᐱ Appendix 9: Informed Consent

T he details of gaining informed consent, from a patient, differ between hospitals (and Trusts), but the main requirements for gaining consent are defined by the General Medical Council, and doctors are expected to comply with those requirements, a selection of which follows:

⚓ Give the patient the information they want or need in a way they can understand.

⚓ Be honest and open and act with integrity.

⚓ You are personally accountable for your professional practice and must always be prepared to justify your decisions and actions.

⚓ Listen to the patient, and respect their views about their health

⚓ The doctor and patient make an assessment of the patient's condition, taking into account the patient's medical history, views, experience and knowledge.

⚓ The doctor must provide the patient with information about the potential benefits, risks and burdens, and the likelihood of success, for each option; this should include information, if available, about whether the benefits or risks are affected by which organisation or doctor is chosen to provide care.

🪲 The patient has a right to seek a second opinion.

🪲 You (doctor) should check whether the patient has understood the information they have been given, and whether or not they would like more information before making a decision.

🪲 Involve other members of the healthcare team in discussions with the patient, if appropriate.

🪲 Give the patient time to reflect, before and after they make a decision, especially if the information is complex, or what you are proposing involves significant risks.

🪲 In order to have effective discussions with the patient about risk, you must identify the adverse outcomes that may result from the proposed options. This includes the potential outcome of taking no action. Risks can take a number of forms, but will usually be:

☞ Side effects

☞ Complications

☞ Failure of an intervention to achieve the desired aim

🪲 Risks can vary from common but minor side effects, to rare but serious adverse outcomes, possibly resulting in permanent disability or death.

🪲 In assessing the risk to an individual patient, you must consider the nature of the patient's condition, their general health and other circumstances. These are variable.

🪲 You must tell the patient if an investigation or treatment might result in an adverse outcome, even if the likelihood is very small.

🔱 You must use the patient's medical records or a consent form to record the key elements of your discussion with the patient. This should include the information you discussed, any specific requests by the patient, any written, visual or audio information given to the patient, and details of any decisions that were made.

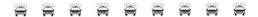

📖 Final Comments

NHS *Dirty Secrets* has shown how the cover-up culture of the NHS is a threat to the safety of patients, and is made real by what I call the *NHS Triad of Cover-up of Factors*. The first factor, **maskirovka**, is described as being the foundation of the cover-up culture, whose object is to conceal or disguise the true state of any particular issue that might prove detrimental to the image and job security of relevant NHS officials, or damaging to the image of the government of the day, and its ministers.

The second factor, **propaganda**, is the set of techniques used to attempt to influence the public's understanding and opinions of how the NHS is being managed, towards one that is more positive than it otherwise might be. Propaganda statements are substitutes for information that has been concealed by maskirovka techniques.

The final factor is that of **bullying**, which is how the NHS manages to dissuade employees from revealing the truth about issues that may have been concealed by maskirovka, or misrepresented by propaganda.

To support the NHS cover-up culture, the NHS must employ the appropriately tyrannical people who provide that support, and those people have to be given the power with which to enforce the cover-up culture over other staff, through their willingness to bully them into acquiescence. The power to bully others is made possible by seniority, so the cover-up supporters tend to achieve promotion more quickly than those who are not so compliant with the cover-up culture. Clearly, then, promotion in the NHS is not directly related to ability or merit but, instead, promotion and ability are often inversely proportional. This is why there are so many falsely qualified bullying managers and team leaders in the NHS, and the bullying and intimidation of more junior employees is how those bullies preserve their jobs.

A significant consequence of the NHS cover-up culture concerns that of there being no opportunity for the rest of the service to learn from mistakes made by another part of the service. Safety, then, is degraded by the practice of covering-up mistakes. Degraded safety, in turn, stimulates the more conscientious members of the NHS workforce to disclose those safety issues by drawing attention to them with protected disclosures (whistleblowing) to appropriate government agencies. Making such disclosures then results in more reflexive bullying from the whistleblower's employer, usually resulting in counter accusations of one sort or another. The cover-up cycle is thus:

♟ **Increased covering-up requires increased bullying to deter whistleblowers; increased maskirovka to prevent the public from discovering the issue being covered-up, and increased propaganda to provide the public with an alternative "truth" about the matter. The end result is a reduction in patient safety.**

♟ **A decrease in patient safety increases the probability of** whistleblowing.

🕱 **Whistleblowing weakens the cover-up culture.**

🕱 **A weakened cover-up culture is strengthened by increased propaganda, more bullying, more cover-ups, and more employment and promotion of supporters of the cover-up culture.**

So it goes on and repeats. The relationship between the NHS cover-up culture and degraded safety is clear, and is proven every time a new NHS cover-up scandal is made public. Intuitively, the public might assume that NHS Directors, Managers, and clinical safety "tzars" (or safety "champions") should be proactive with respect to understanding the principles and legal aspects of safety, so that they might better present themselves when confronted with interrogations about safety attitudes and incidents - but they don't. The ignorance about the theory and practice of safety regimes, amongst NHS professionals, is criminally low and, when considering the issue of the *Precautionary Principle*, ignorance is absolute. I have had conversations with senior clinical staff, who have been appointed departmental safety "champions", about how particular behaviours fail to comply with the *Precautionary Principle*, and have been met, every time, with confused silence. NHS "safety champions" do not understand safety - exceptions, if any, are rare.

By appointing someone, such as a senior nurse, to be a safety "champion", a manager can boast that safety is a top priority and, as way of proof, they can claim that their department has a safety expert. The truth is that safety "champion" appointments are made for propaganda purposes only, and there is no substance to them.

In total, employment in the NHS is characterised by behaviours and practices that produce inequalities, and oppression of specific groups. The behaviours and practices relate to discrimination and favouritism for the two different groups (for or against covering up); inequalities are illustrated by career advancement and job protection for the supporters of the cover-up culture, and oppression is used to punish whistleblowers, or to deter those who might be tempted to follow the whistleblowing path. Interestingly, the above description of how the NHS is characterised intersects with the United Nations definition of an **oppressive regime**:

> The laws, customs, or practices that systematically produce inequalities, and oppress specific groups within a society.

NHS Dirty Secrets has exposed many of the worst features of the NHS, including those "rogue" employees and officials who are responsible for maintaining the cover-up culture, and its consequent degradation of safe patient care.

There will, inevitably, be many supporters and beneficiaries of the NHS cover-up culture who will object to the message that this book gives. Some of those people may make the predictable accusations that some of the things I have written have been included to add a degree of sensationalism, with the aim of selling more books. My response to those people is to paraphrase Mandy Rice-Davies, by saying "They would say that, wouldn't they?".

Readers should not assume that this is the whole story of the NHS, and should not be deterred from using its services, because, for most NHS patients, the service they receive is as good as many other of the world's national health services.

The "rogue" incompetents, fraudsters, sex predators, bullies, drug addicts and the like, are the few rotten apples in a large basket of apples. The NHS does employ many highly competent, well educated, and caring people, including some of the world's best doctors, nurses, and allied professionals, who are genuinely concerned about the outcomes of their patients, so nobody should be frightened of using the NHS. Unfortunately, when failures occur, and they occur frequently, the NHS tends to deny or hide those mistakes, preferring, instead, to avoid remedying and learning from mistakes, because its leaders prefer to take the road of individual and collective career protection, and keep the public ignorant of NHS Dirty Secrets.

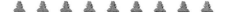

Printed in Great Britain
by Amazon

77044413R00203